Cardiopulmonary Anatomy and Physiology Essentials for Respiratory Care

Workbook

NOTICE TO THE READER

Publisher does not warrant or guarantee any of the products described herein or perform any independent analysis in connection with any of the product information contained herein. Publisher does not assume, and expressly disclaims, any obligation to obtain and include information other than that provided to it by the manufacturer.

The reader is expressly warned to consider and adopt all safety precautions that might be indicated by the activities described herein and to avoid all potential hazards. By following the instructions contained herein, the reader willingly assumes all risks in connection with such instructions.

The publisher makes no representations or warranties of any kind, including but not limited to, the warranties of fitness for particular purpose or merchantability, nor are any such representations implied with respect to the material set forth herein, and the publisher takes no responsibility with respect to such material. The publisher shall not be liable for any special, consequential or exemplary damages resulting, in whole or in part, from the readers' use of, or reliance upon, this material.

For information, address Delmar Publishers Inc.
3 Columbia Circle, Box 15-015
Albany, NY 12212

printed in the United States of America
published simultaneously in Canada
by Nelson Canada,
a division of The Thomson Corporation

1 2 3 4 5 6 7 8 9 10 XXX 99 98 97 96 95 94 93

Library of Congress Catalog Card Number: 92-14625
ISBN: 0-8273-5006-6

INTRODUCTION

This workbook is designed to enhance the learner's understanding, retention, and clinical application of the material presented in the textbook. The questions in the workbook parallel (in a step-by-step fashion) the information presented in the textbook. The student is asked to do such things as: label and color illustrations, fill in the blanks, define terms, match answers, calculate equations, and write short answers. Answers to the questions, with page references to the textbook (a remedial-loop mechanism), appear at the end of the workbook.

The completed study questions serve as an excellent study tool to review and prepare for chapter quizzes and exams. This workbook also gives the reader an opportunity to evaluate the degree of mastery of the material presented in the text. Although answering 75% of the questions correctly is considered an acceptable mastery level, study and review should continue until greater than 90% has been achieved. The student may wish to copy and maintain unanswered questions of various sections of the workbook for reuse and periodic self-assessment.

Terry Des Jardins

CONTENTS

CHAPTER ONE
THE ANATOMY OF THE RESPIRATORY SYSTEM

SECTION A

1. Label and color the following structures of the upper airway:

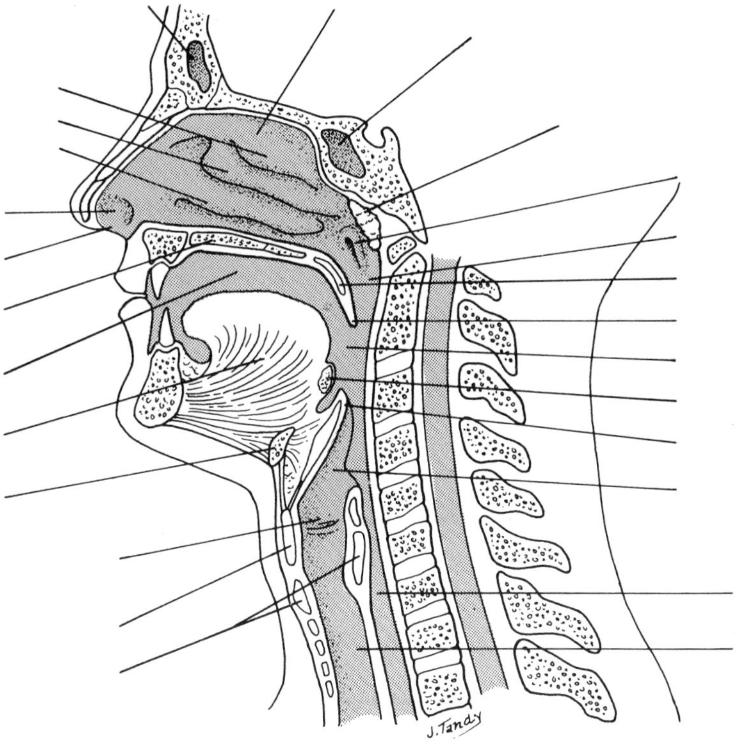

Sagittal section of human head, showing the upper airway.

2. The primary function(s) of the upper airway are:

   a. ______________________________

   ____

   b. ______________________________

   ____

   c. ______________________________

   ____

3. The primary functions of the nose is to do the following to inspired air:

   a. ____________________

   b. ____________________

   c. ____________________

4. Label and color the following structures that form the outer portion of the nose:

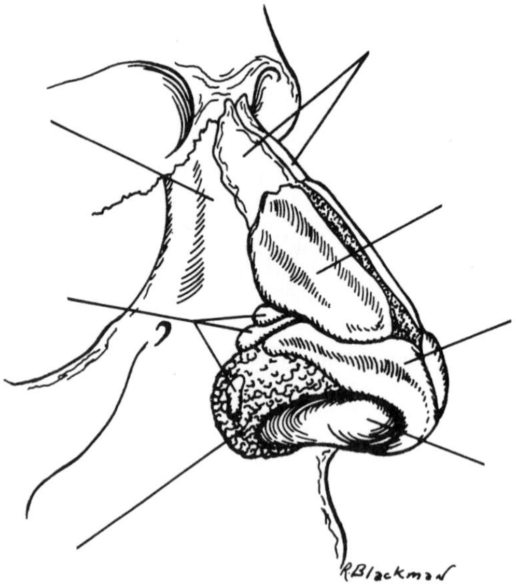

Structure of the nose.

5. Label and color the following structures of the internal portion of the nose:

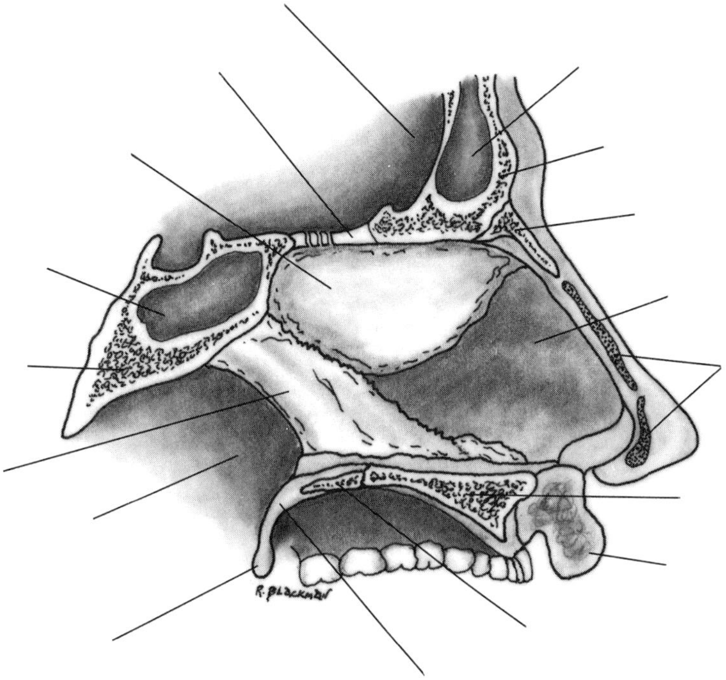

Sagittal section through the nose, showing the parts of the nasal septum.

6. ______________________________ epithelium lines the posterior two-thirds of the nasal cavity.

7. List the three bony protrusions in the nasal cavity that increase the contact time between the inspired air and the warm, moist surface of the nasal cavity?

a. ______________________________

b. ______________________________

c. ______________________________

8. Label and color the following sinuses of the skull:

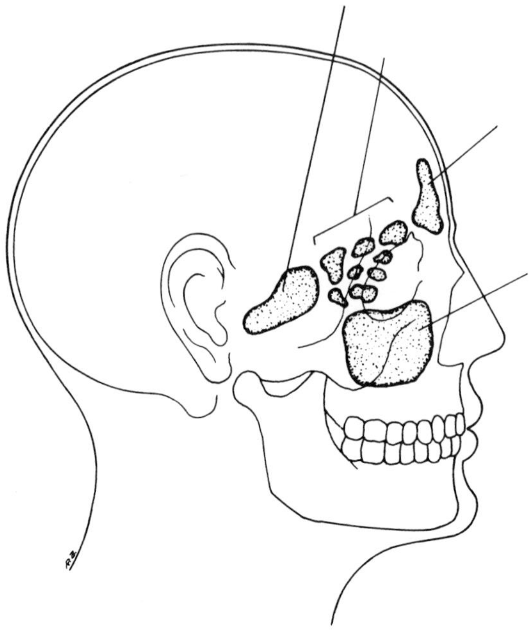

Lateral view of head, showing sinuses. Adapted from Short, *Essential Anatomies: Oral and Head/Neck,* 1987 by Delmar Publishers Inc.

9. The ______________________ muscle elevates the soft palate.

10. The oral cavity is lined with ______________________ epithelium.

11. The **palatine arches** are composed of the ______________ arch and the ______________ arch.

12. The **nasopharynx** is lined with ______________________ epithelium.

13. The ______________ serves to equalize the pressure between the nasopharynx and the middle ear.

14. The **oropharynx** is lined with ______________________ epithelium.

15. The **laryngopharynx** is lined with ______________________ epithelium.

16. Label and color the following structures of the oral cavity.

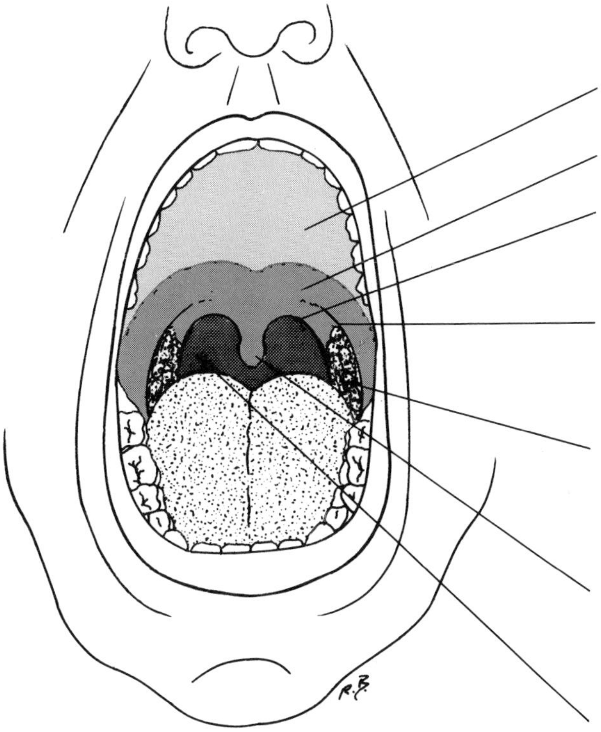

Oral cavity.

SECTION B

1. Functionally, the **larynx**:

   a. ______________________________

   ____

   ____

   b. ______________________________

   ____

   ____

   c. ______________________________

   ____

   ____

2. Label and color the following cartilages of the larynx:

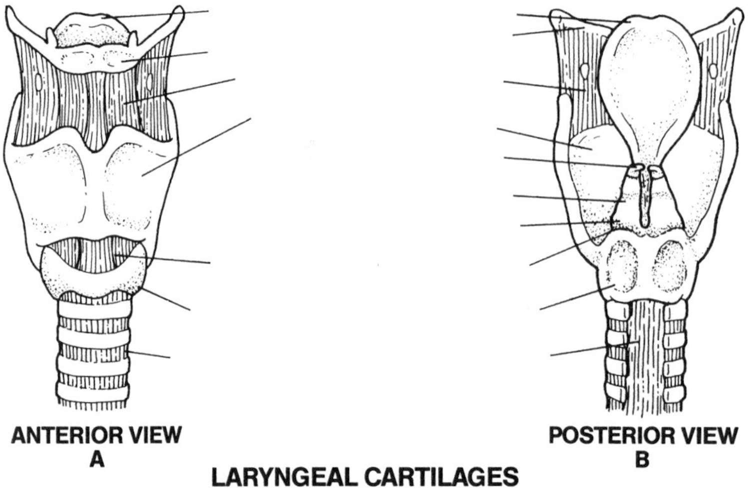

Cartilages of the larynx.

3. Label and color the structures observed in the superior view of the vocal folds:

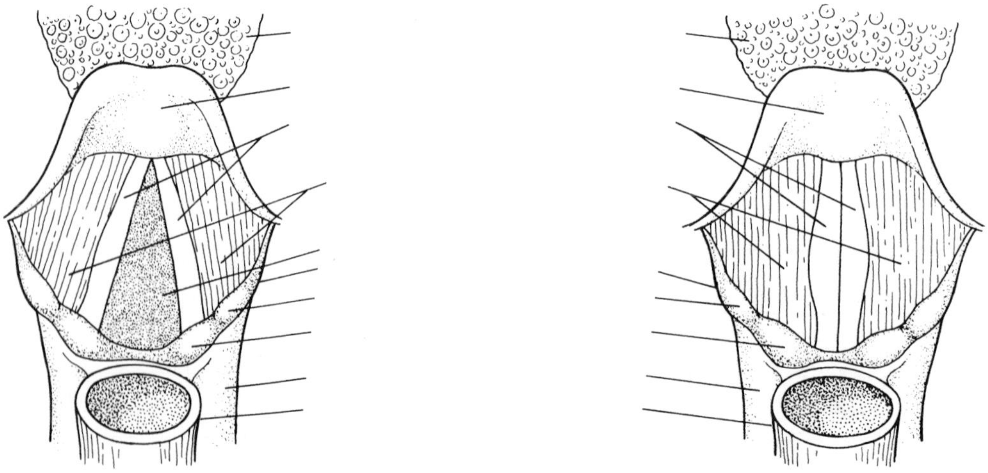

Superior view of vocal folds (cords).

4. The elastic tissue that form the medial border of each vocal fold is called the ______________________________.

5. Anteriorly, the vocal cords attach to the posterior surface of the ______________________________.

6. The space between the vocal cords is called the ______________________ or the ______________________.

7. Above the vocal cords, the laryngeal mucosa is composed of ______________________________ epithelium.

8. Below the vocal cords, the laryngeal mucosa is lined with ______________________________ epithelium.

9. An expiratory effort against a closed glottis (e.g., during physical work such as lifting or pushing) is known as ______________ ______________________.

10. Label and color the following **intrinsic muscles** of the larynx:

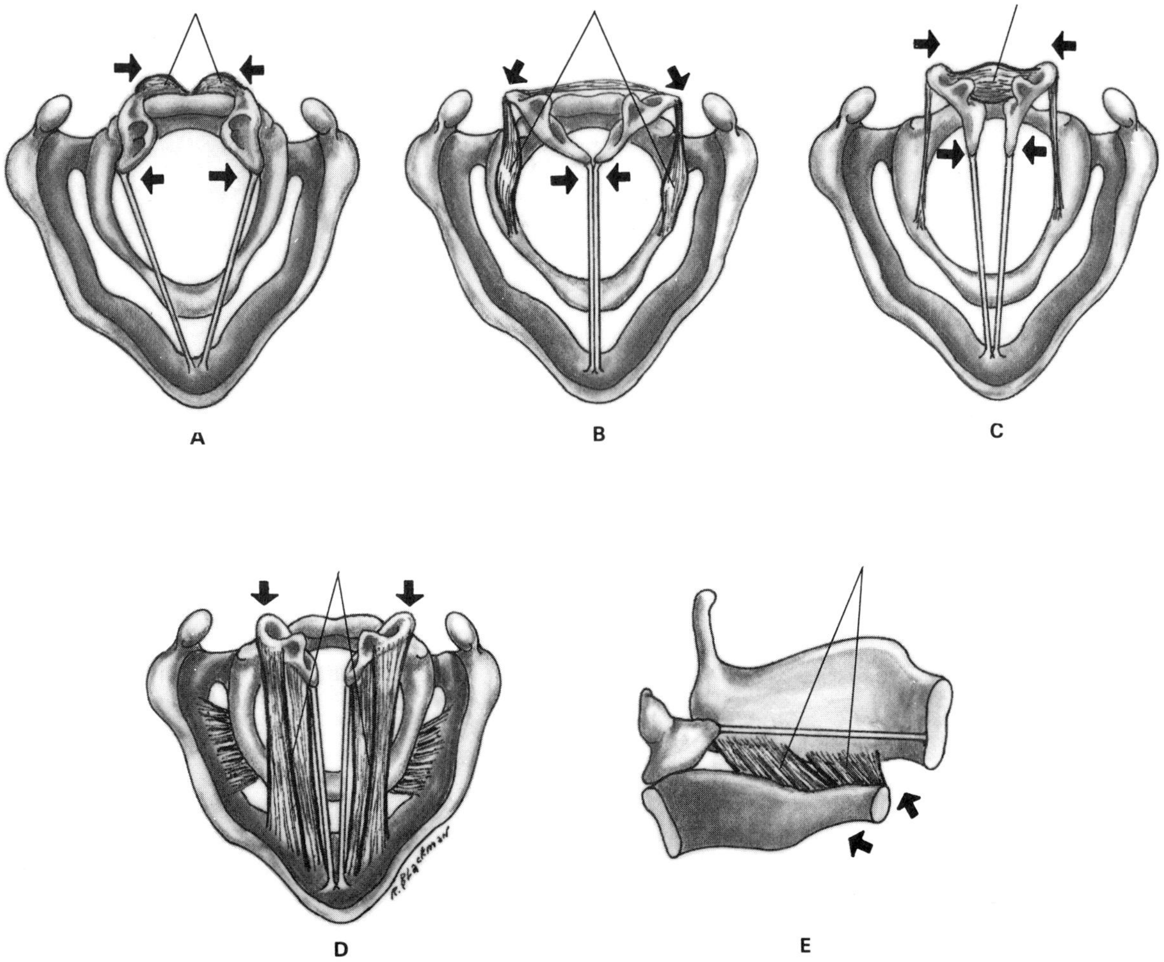

Intrinsic laryngeal muscles.

11. Label and color the following **extrinsic laryngeal** muscles:

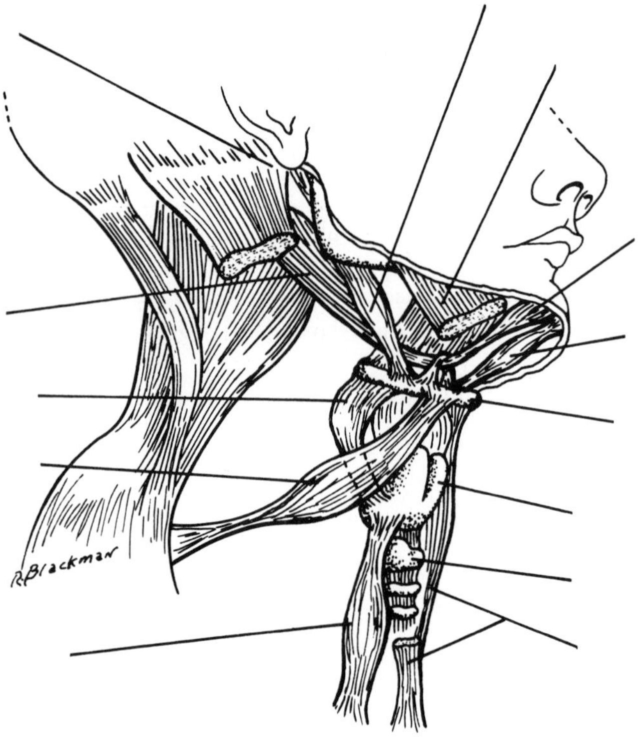

Extrinsic laryngeal muscles. Adapted from Short, *Essential Anatomies: Oral and Head/Neck,* © 1987 by Delmar Publishers Inc.

SECTION C

1. The tracheobronchial tree is composed of the following three layers:

   a. ____________________

   b. ____________________

   c. ____________________

2. The epithelial lining of the tracheobronchial tree is mainly composed of ____________________ epithelium.

3. Most of the mucous that lines the lumen of the tracheobronchial tree is produced by the ____________________.

4. The two distinct layers of the mucous blanket are the (1)____________________ and the (2) ____________________.

5. Label and color the following section of epithelial lining of the tracheobronchial tree:

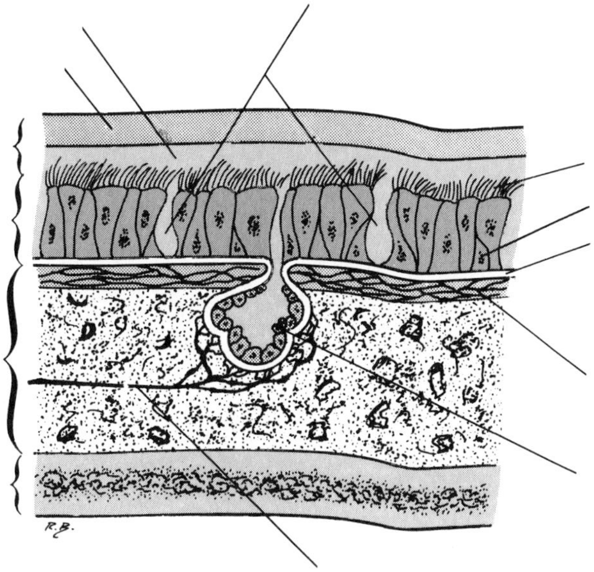

Epithelial lining of the tracheobronchial tree.

6. List factors that are known to slow the rate of the mucociliary transport mechanism

a. ______________________________

b. ______________________________

c. ______________________________

d. ______________________________

e. ______________________________

f. ______________________________

g. ______________________________

h. ______________________________

i. ______________________________

7. List five chemical mediators of inflammation secreted by the mast cell

   a. ____________________

   b. ____________________

   c. ____________________

   d. ____________________

   e. ____________________

8. The adult trachea is about ____ to ____ cm long and ____ to ____ cm in diameter.

9. The bifurcation of the trachea is known as the ____________________.

10. In the adult, the right main stem bronchus branches off the vertical trachea at about a __________ degree angle; the left main stem bronchus forms a _______ to _______ angle with the vertical trachea.

11. **Canals of Lambert** are found in the ____________________ of the tracheobronchial tree.

12. From the trachea to the terminal bronchioles, the total cross-sectional area of the tracheobronchial tree progressively

    ____________________.

13. The bronchial arteries nourish the tracheobronchial tree down to, and including, the ____________________.

14. In addition to the tracheobronchial tree, the bronchial arteries nourish the ____________________

    ____

    ____

    ____

15. Approximately one-third of the bronchial venous blood returns to the right atrium by way of the ____________________

    ____

16. About two-thirds of the bronchial venous blood empties into the pulmonary circulation by means of ____________________

    ____

SECTION D

1. The anatomic structures distal to the terminal bronchioles consist of the:

   a. ____________________ bronchioles

   b. ____________________ ducts

   c. ____________________ sacs

2. Using the following schematic drawing, label the following anatomic structures distal to the terminal bronchiole:

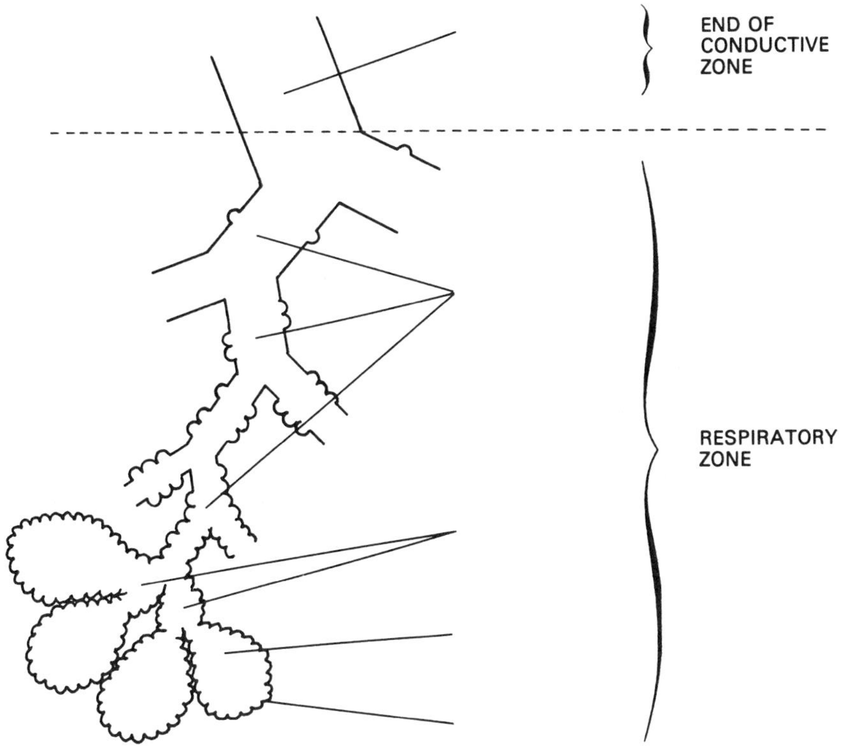

Schematic drawing of the anatomic structures distal to the terminal bronchioles; collectively, these are referred to as the primary lobule.

3. Label and color the following components of the alveolar-capillary network:

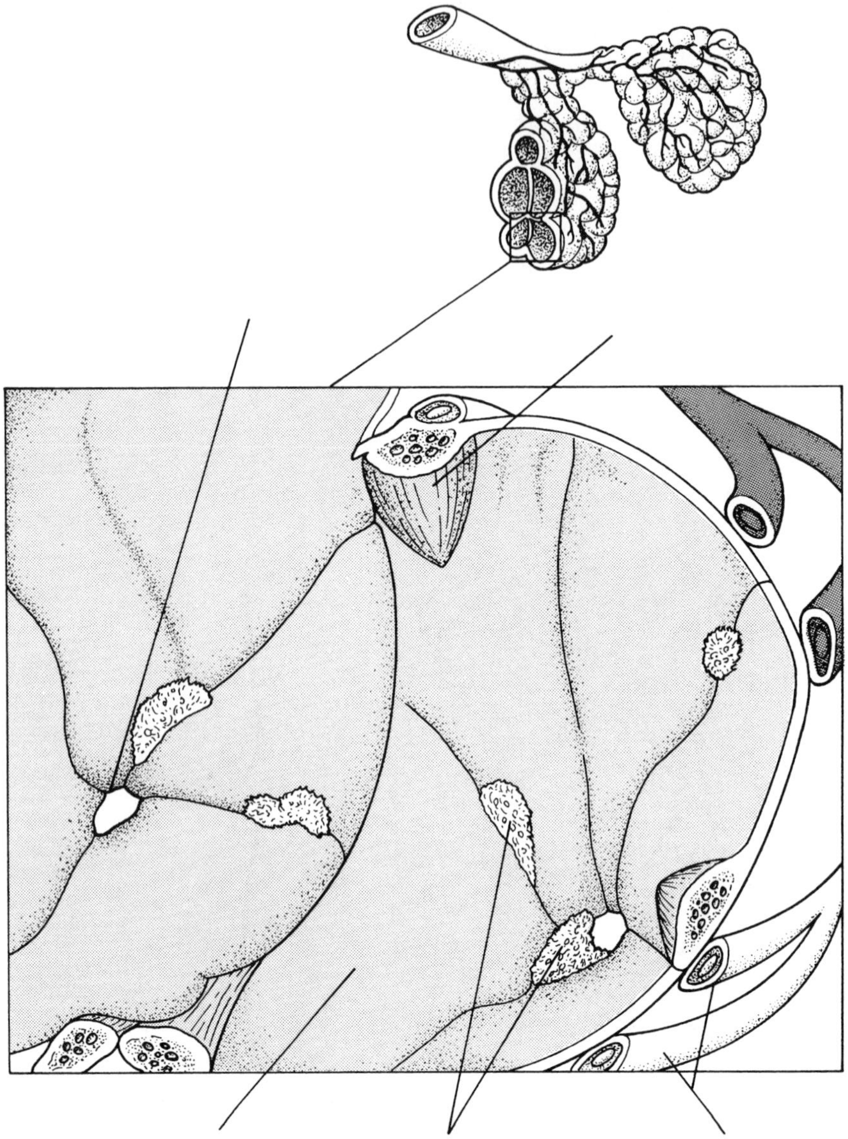

Alveolar-capillary network.

4. In the adult lung, there are approximately ______ million alveoli.

5. The average surface area of the adult lung is ______ square meters.

6. A **primary lobules** consist of what structures distal to a single terminal bronchiole?

____

____

7. There are approximately ____________________ primary lobules in the lung.

8. Synonyms for primary lobules are:

a. ______________________________

b. ______________________________

c. ______________________________

d. ______________________________

9. The **Type I cell** found in the alveolar epithelium is also called

a ______________________________.

10. The **Type II cell** found in the alveolar epithelium is also called

a ______________________________.

11. The Type I cells form about ________ % of the alveolar substance.

12. The ______________ cells are believed to be the primary source of pulmonary surfactant.

13. Small holes in the walls of the interalveolar septa are called

______________________________.

14. The ______________________________ play a major role in removing foreign particles that are deposited within the acini.

15. The two major compartments of the interstitium are the____________________

and the ________________________.

SECTION E

1. Using the following schematic drawing, label and color the components of the major blood vessels:

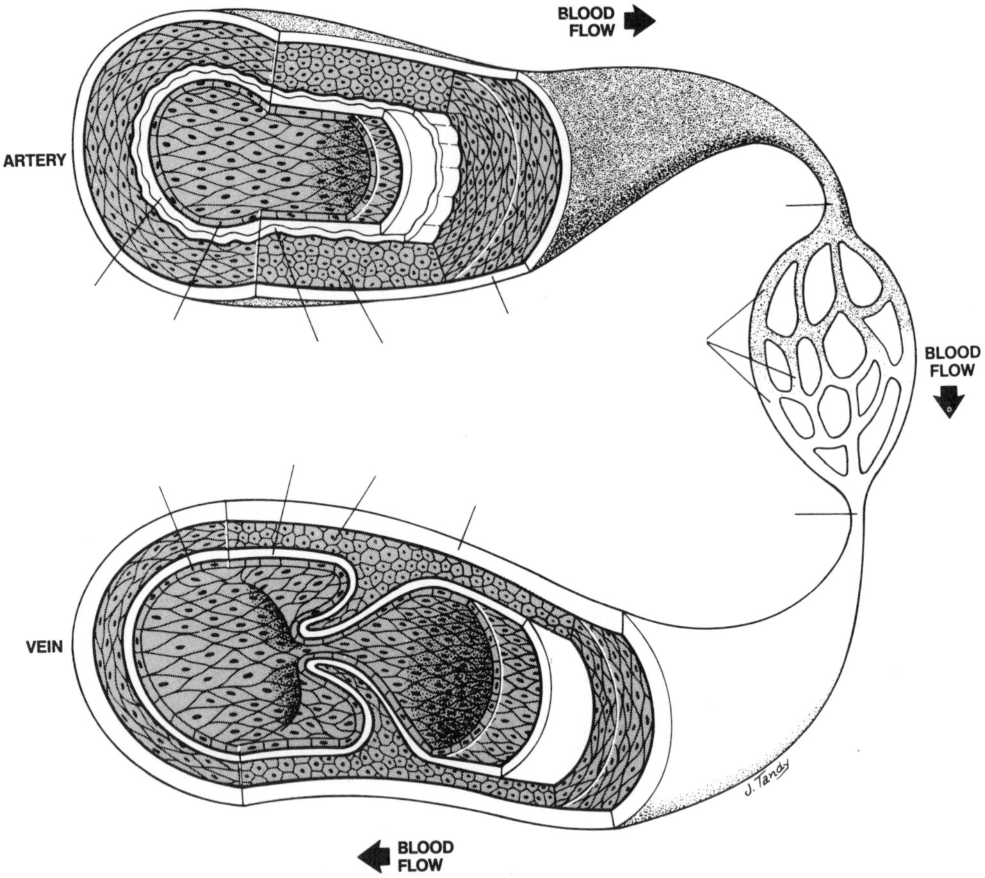

Schematic drawing of the components of the major blood vessels.

2. The arterioles play an important role in the distribution and regulation of blood and are called the ______________________________ vessels.

3. The walls of the pulmonary capillaries are less than ________________ thick and the external diameter is about ____________________.

4. Because the veins are capable of collecting a large amount of blood with very little pressure change, the veins are called ____________________________ vessels.

5. Superficially, lymphatic vessels are found around the lung just beneath the ______________________________________.

6. Within the lungs, the lymphatic vessels arise from the ______________ ____.

7. Label the following lymph nodes associated with the trachea and the right and left main stem bronchi:

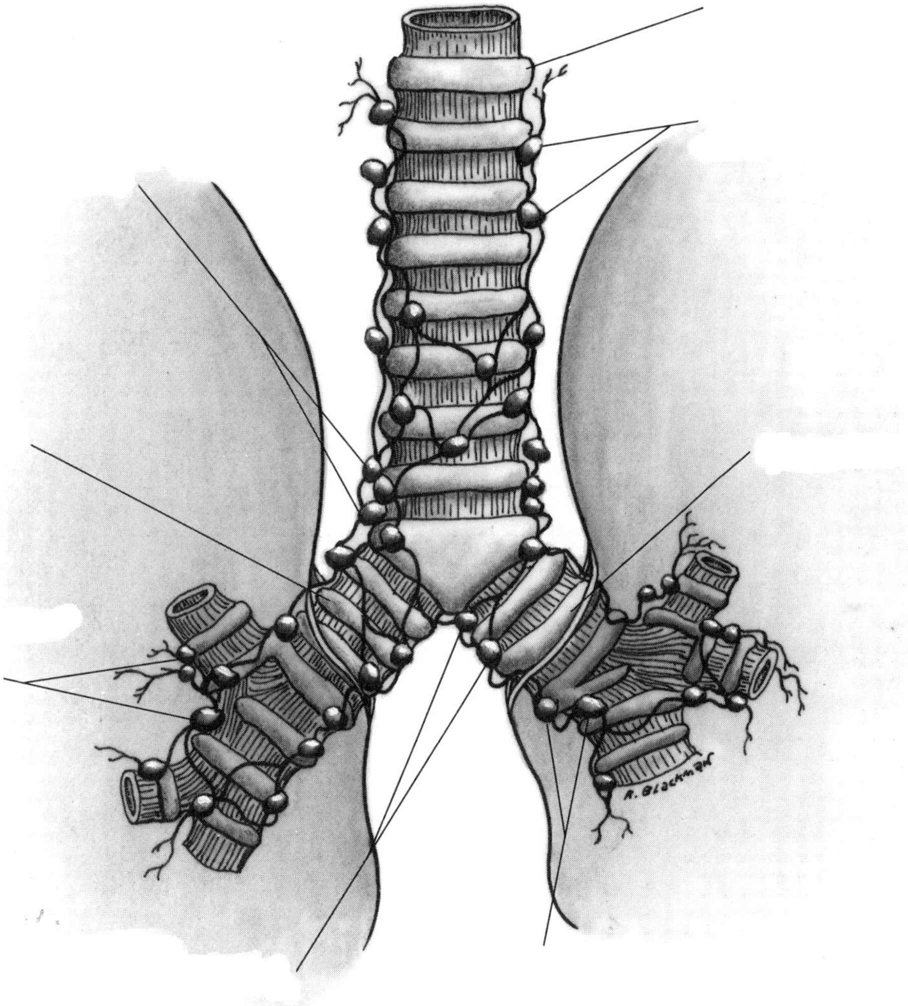

Lymph nodes associated with the trachea and the right and left main stem bronchi.

8. The smooth muscle that surrounds the bronchi and arterioles is controlled by the ____.

9. Compare and contrast the effects of the sympathetic and parasympathetic nervous system on the following effector sites:

TABLE 1–2. Some Effects of Autonomic Nervous System Activity

EFFECTOR SITE	SYMPATHETIC NERVOUS SYSTEM	PARASYMPATHETIC NERVOUS SYSTEM
Heart		
Bronchial smooth muscle		
Bronchial glands		
Salivary glands		
Stomach		
Intestines		
Eye		

10. When the sympathetic nervous system is activated, ______________________ or ______________________ neural transmitters are released.

11. When the **beta$_2$** receptors are stimulated, the bronchial smooth muscles ______________________.

12. When the **alpha receptors** are stimulated, the smooth muscles of the arterioles ______________________.

13. When the parasympathetic nervous system is activated, the neural transmitter ______________________ is released.

SECTION F

1. The apex of the lungs rise to about the level of the _________ rib.

2. Anteriorly, the base of the lungs external to about the level of the _____________ rib, and posteriorly to about the level of the _____ _____________ rib.

3. At the center of the mediastinal border, the right and left main stem bronchi, blood vessels, lymph vessels, and various nerves enter and exit the lungs through the _____________.

4. In the right lung, the **oblique fissure** extends from the _______ _______________ to the _____________________ borders.

5. In the right lung, the **horizontal fissure** extends horizontally from the ___________________ to about the level of the _____________ costal cartilage.

6. In the left lung, the **oblique fissure** extends from the ___________ to the ___________________ borders of the lung.

7. Label the following structures of the anterior portion of the lungs:

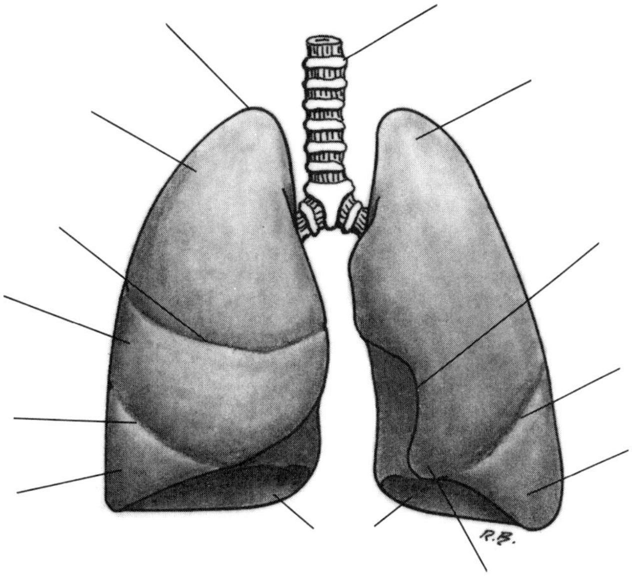

Anterior view of the lungs.

8. Label the following structures of the medial portion of the lungs:

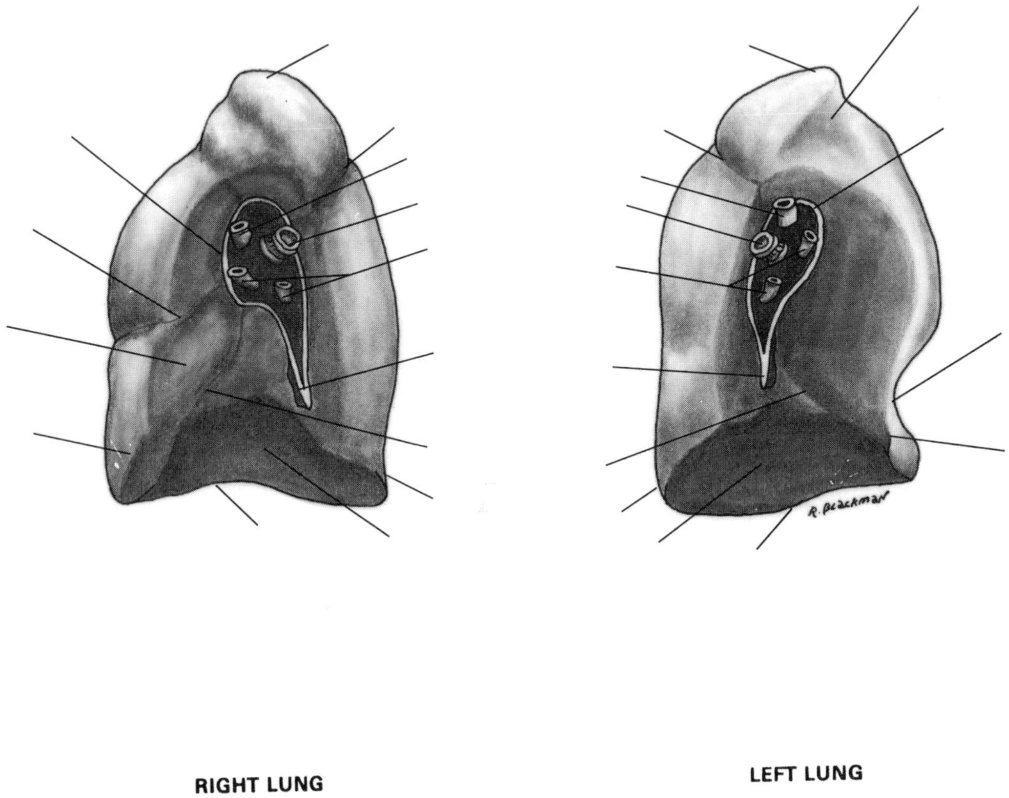

Medial view of the lungs.

9. Match the number of the lung segments shown in the box to the different views of the lung. Content retention is also enhanced when the lung segments are colored.

RIGHT LUNG		LEFT LUNG	
UPPER LOBE		UPPER LOBE	
		UPPER DIVISION	
APICAL	1	APICAL/POSTERIOR	1&2
POSTERIOR	2		
ANTERIOR	3	ANTERIOR	3
MIDDLE LOBE		LOWER DIVISION (LINGULAR)	
LATERAL	4	SUPERIOR LINGULA	4
MEDIAL	5	INFERIOR LINGULA	5
LOWER LOBE		LOWER LOBE	
SUPERIOR	6	SUPERIOR	6
MEDIAL BASAL	7	ANTERIOR MEDIAL	7&8
ANTERIOR BASAL	8	LATERAL BASAL	9
LATERAL BASAL	9	POSTERIOR BASAL	10
POSTERIOR BASAL	10		

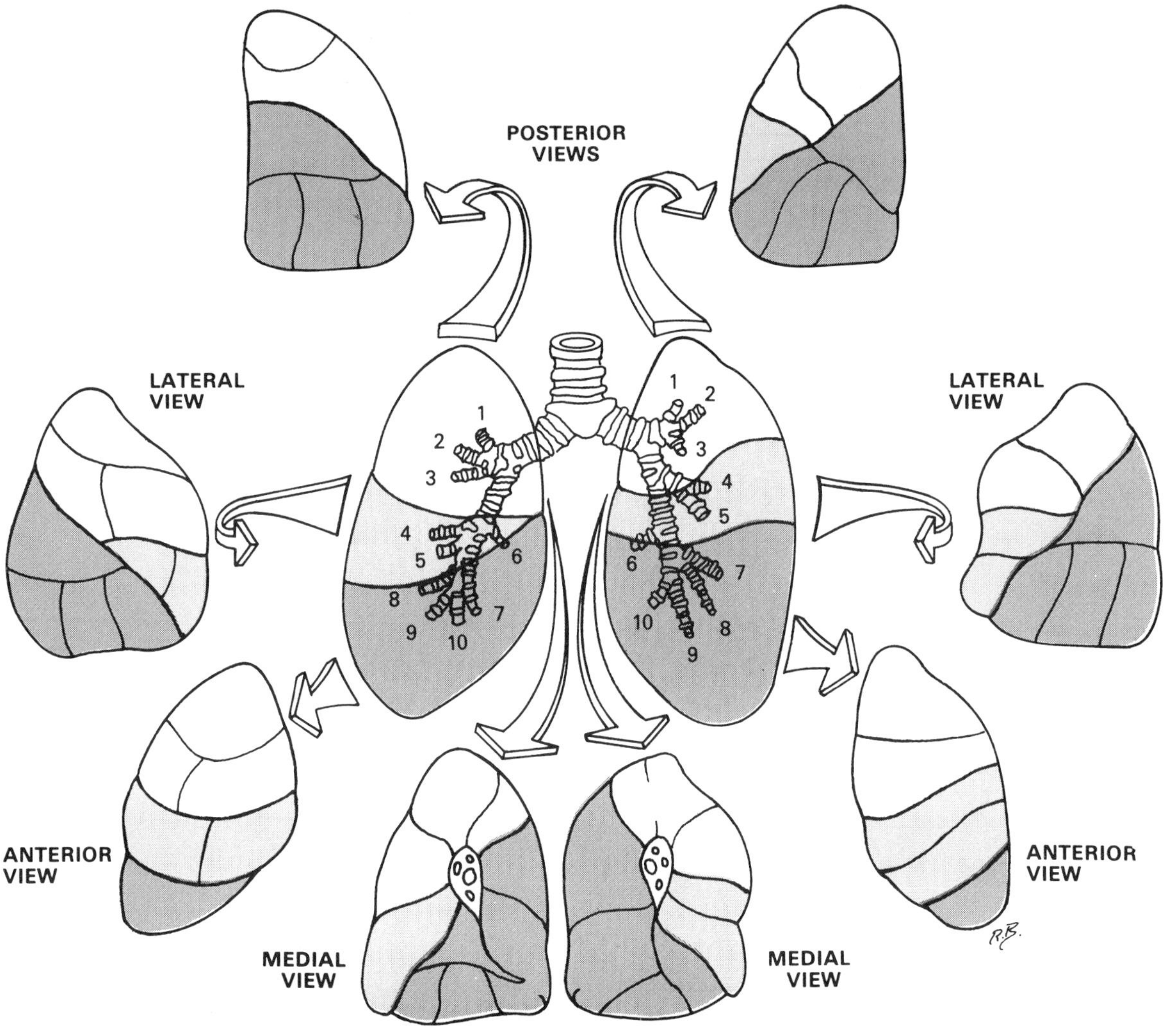

Lung segments. Although the segment subdivisions of the right and left lungs are similar, there are some slight anatomic differences, which are noted by combined names and numbers. Because of these slight variations, some workers consider that, technically, there are only eight segments in the left lung and that the apical-posterior segment in number 1 and the anteromedial is number 6.

10. List the anatomic structures that are contained in, or pass through, the **mediastinum.**

____

____

____

11. The ______________ pleura is firmly attached to the outer surface of each lung.

12. The ______________ pleura lines the inside of the thoracic walls.

13. The potential space between the pleural membranes is called the

______________________.

14. List the three major structures that compose the sternum.

a. ______________________

b. ______________________

c. ______________________

15. The first seven ribs are called the ______________________.

16. Ribs eight, nine, and ten are referred to as the ______________ ribs.

17. Ribs eleven and twelve are called the ______________ ribs.

18. Label the following components of the thorax:

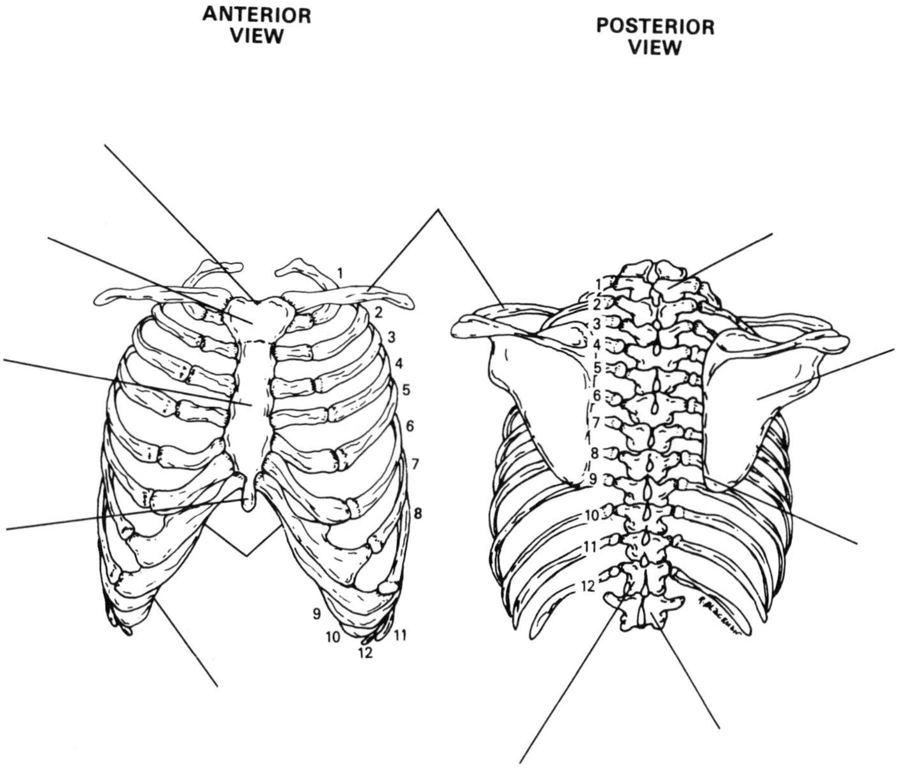

The thorax.

19. Label the following components of the intercostal space:

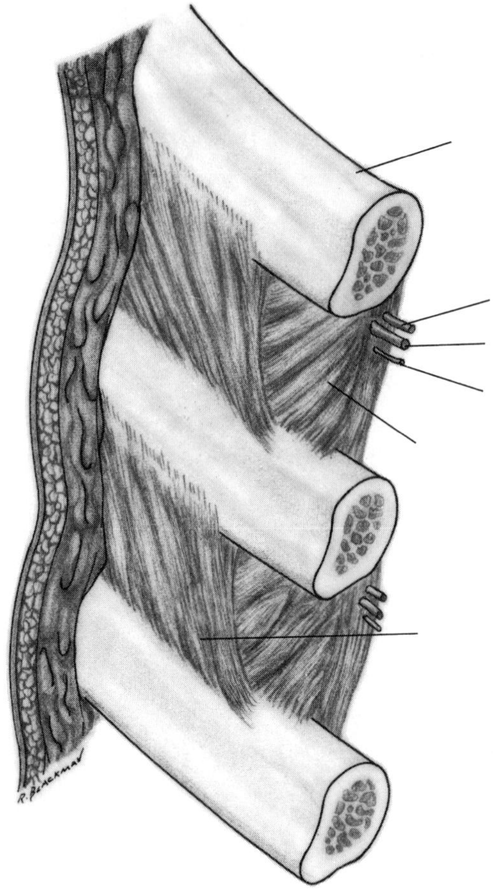

The intercostal space.

SECTION G

1. Each hemidiaphragm merges together at the midline into a broad connective sheet called the ________________________________.

2. List the structures that pierce the diaphragm. ________________

____

____

3. The ____________________ nerves supply the primary motor innervation to each hemidiaphragm.

4. When used as accessory muscles for inspiration, the **scalene muscles** elevate the ______________ and ________________ ribs.

5. When used as accessory muscles of inspiration, the **sterno-cleidomastoid muscles** elevate the ____________________.

6. When used as accessory muscles of inspiration, the **pectoralis major muscles** elevate the _______________ causing an increased ______________________ diameter.

7. Normally, the **trapezius** rotates the ______________, raises the ____________, and abducts and flexes the ______________.

8. During inspiration, the **external intercostal muscles** pull the ribs _____________ and _____________.

9. Label and color the following accessory muscles of expiration:

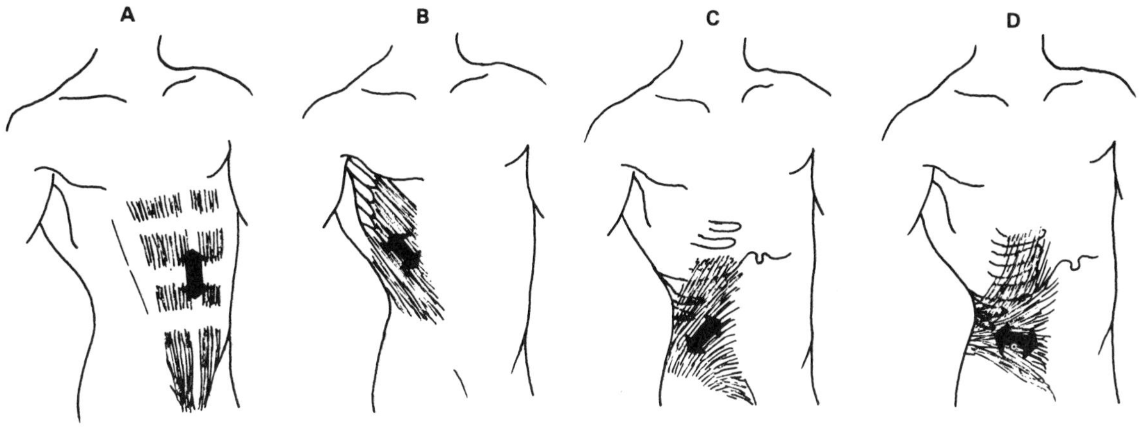

Accessory muscles of expiration.

10. During exhalation, the **internal intercostal muscles** pull the ribs _______________ and _______________.

Chapter Two
Ventilation

SECTION A

1. The pressure difference between two points in a tube or vessel is called the ______________________________.

2. The barometric pressure difference between the mouth pressure and alveolar pressure is called the ______________________________.

3. The difference between the alveolar pressure and the pleural pressure is called the ______________________________.

4. The difference between the alveolar pressure and the body surface pressure is called the ______________________________.

5. If the gas pressure at the beginning of a vessel is 12 mm Hg and the pressure at the other end of the same vessel is 7 mm Hg, what is the driving pressure?

   Answer________________

6. If the P_{alv} is 751 mm Hg and the P_m is 758 mm Hg, what is the P_{ta}?

   Answer________________

7. If the P_{pl} is 752 mm Hg and the P_{alv} is 748 mm Hg, what is the P_{tp}?

Answer_________________

8. If the P_{alv} is 751 mm Hg and the P_{bs} is 757 mm Hg, what is the P_{tt}?

Answer_________________

9. During inspiration, the thoracic volume increases and the intrapleural and intra-alveolar pressures ___________________.

10. During expiration, the intra-alveolar pressure is (_____greater; _____lower) than the barometric pressure.

11. During a normal expiration, the intrapleural pressure is always (_____above; _____below) the barometric pressure.

12. The normal intrapleural pressure change is about _______ to _______ cm H_2O pressure, or _______ to _______ mm Hg.

13. The term **static** refers to ____________________________________

____

____

14. The lungs have a natural tendency to (____ collapse; ____ expand).

15. The chest wall has a natural tendency to (____ collapse; ____ expand).

16. The two major static forces of the lungs are:

    1. ____

       ____

    2. ____

       ____

17. **Lung compliance** is defined as the change in lung ____________ per change in ______________.

- -

18. Case:

- Part I

  If an individual generates an intrapleural pressure of -7 cm H_2O during inspiration, and the lungs accept a new volume of 385 ml of air, what is the compliance of the lungs?

  Answer________________

- Part II

  If the same patient, four hours later, generates an intrapleural pressure of -5 cm H_2O during inspiration, and the lungs accept a new volume of 350 ml of air, what is the compliance of the lungs?

Answer________________

- Part III

The lung compliance of the above patient is:

increasing __________ decreasing __________

- -

19. Case:

Ventilator Dependent Patient

- Part I

If a mechanical ventilator generates a +9 cm H_2O pressure during inspiration and the lungs accept a new volume of 450 ml of gas, what is the compliance of the lungs?

Answer__________________

- Part II

If, on the same patient six hours later, the mechanical ventilator generates a +15 cm H_2O pressure and the lungs accept a new volume of 675 ml of gas, what is the compliance of the lungs?

Answer__________________

- Part III

  In comparing the answers of Part I and Part II, the patient's lung compliance is:

  _______ increasing _______ decreasing

- -

20. Under normal resting conditions, the average lung compliance during each breath is approximately ____________________.

21. According to the following volume-pressure curve, if an individual has a resting lung volume of 1500 ml, and generates a negative 25 cm H_2O pressure (in addition to the negative pressure required to maintain the resting lung volume), how many ml of gas will the lungs accommodate (in addition to the resting lung volume)?

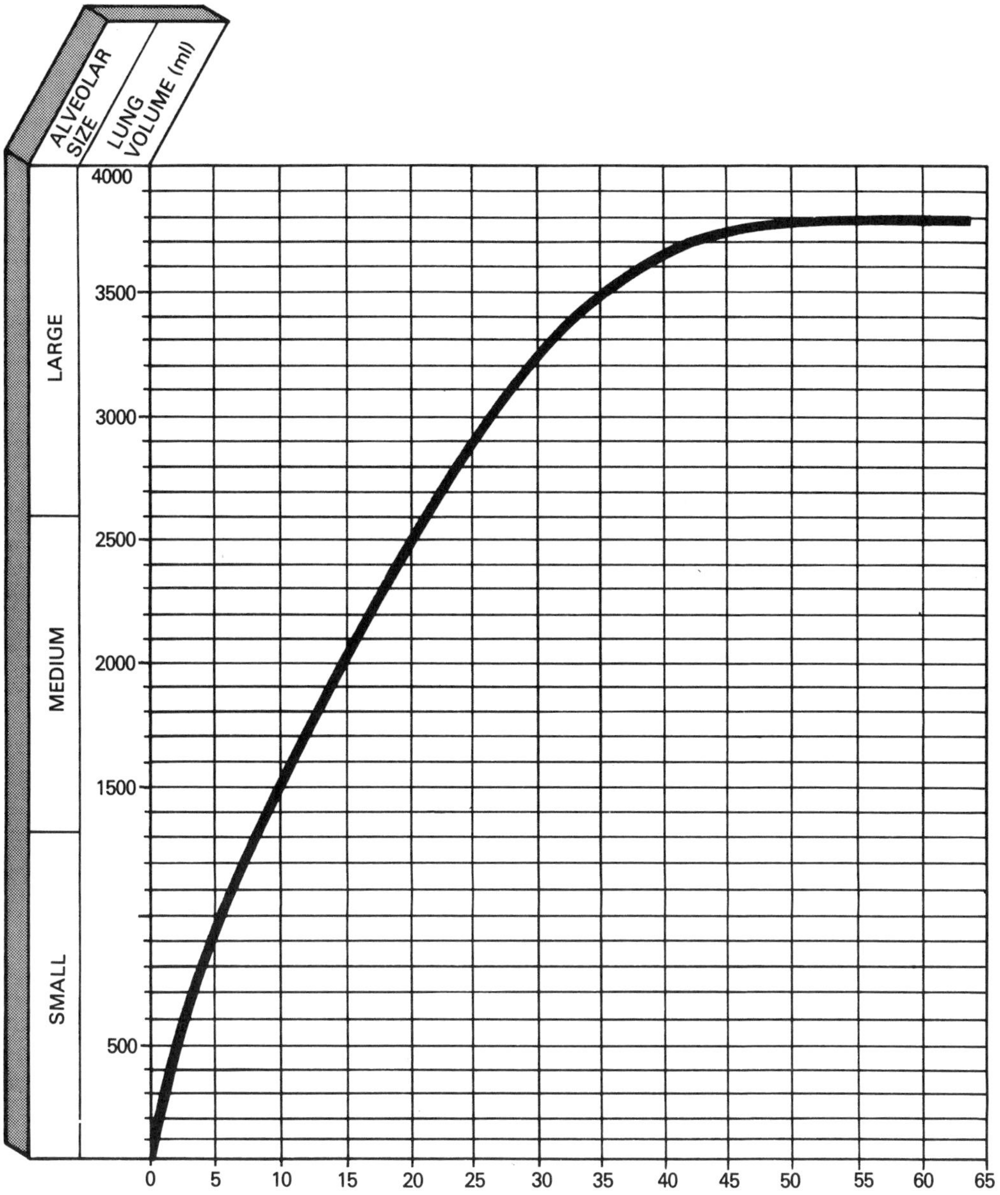

The curve shows that lung compliance progressively decreases as the lungs get larger. For example, note the greater volume change between 5 and 10 cm H_2O (small/medium alveoli) than between 30 and 35 cm H_2O (large alveoli).

Answer________________

22. When lung compliance decreases, the volume-pressure curve moves to the ________________________.

23. When the volume-pressure curve moves to the left, lung compliance is:

    a. increased
    b. decreased
    c. unchanged

24. As the alveoli approach their total filling capacity, lung compliance:

    a. increases
    b. decreases
    c. remains the same

SECTION B

1. **Elastance** is defined as the: ________________________

____

____

____

____

____.

2. In pulmonary physiology, elastance is defined as: ____________

____.

and is expressed as follows:

Elastance =

3. Lungs with high compliance have __________ elastance, and lungs with low compliance have __________ elastance.

4. **Hooke's Law** states that: ____________________________________

____

____

____

____

____

5. When Hooke's Law is applied to the elastic properties of the lungs, _______________ is substituted for length and _________________ is substituted for force.

6. The molecular, cohesive force at the liquid-gas interface is called ___________________________.

7. The liquid film that lines the interior surface of the alveoli has the potential to exert a force of ________________________.

8. When Laplace's Law is applied to a sphere with one liquid-gas interface, the equation is written as follows:

$$P =$$

9. The mathematical arrangement of Laplace's Law shows that the distending pressure of a liquid bubble is

(1)____

____

and (2)_____________________________________

____

10. According to Laplace's Law, as the surface tension of a liquid bubble increases, the distending pressure required to hold the bubble open ______________________________; and as the radius of the bubble increases, the distending pressure ______________________________.

11. When two different size bubbles with the same surface tension are in direct communication the:

    a. larger bubble will empty into the smaller bubble
    b. smaller bubble will empty into the larger bubble
    c. distending pressures in the two bubbles are equal; thus, there is no gas flow between the two bubbles.

12. During the formation of a new bubble, the principles of Laplace's Law do not come into effect until the distending pressure of the liquid sphere goes beyond the ______________________________.

13. As a liquid bubble increases in size, the surface tension:

    a. increases
    b. decreases
    c. remains the same

14. **Pulmonary surfactant** is produced by the ____________________.

15. The surfactant molecule has both a hydrophobic end, which means ____________________, and a hydrophilic end, which means ____________________.

16. In the healthy lung, when the alveolus decreases in size, the amount of surfactant to alveolar surface area ______________. This action causes the alveolar surface tension to ______________.

17. It is estimated that the surface tension of the average alveolus varies from ______________ in the small alveolus to about ______________ in the fully distended alveolus.

18. List some general causes of surfactant deficiency.

    a. ______________________________
    b ______________________________
    c. ______________________________
    d. ______________________________
    e. ______________________________

19. In the healthy lung, both the elastic force and the surface tension force are (____ low; ____ high) in the small alveolus.

SECTION C

1. The term **dynamic** is defined as the:______________________________

____

2. In the lungs, dynamic refers to:__________________________________

____

____

3. When **Poiseuille's Law** is arranged for flow $\dot{V}$, it is written as follows:

$$\dot{V} =$$

4. According to Poiseuille's Law, and assuming all other variables remain the same, as the:

   a. pressure increases, flow (____ increases; ____ decreases)

   b. length of a tube decreases, flow (____ increases; ____ decreases)

   c. radius of a tube increases, flow (____ increases; ____ decreases)

   d. viscosity decreases, flow (____ increases; ____ decreases)

5. POISEUILLE'S LAW EQUATIONS

   Assuming all other variables remain the same:

   a. If the radius of a tube, which has gas flowing through it at 32 liters per minute, is reduced by 50% of its original size, what will be the new gas flow through the tube?

   Answer: ________________________

b. If the radius of a tube, which has gas flowing through it at 28 liters per minute, is reduced by 16%, what will be the new gas flow through the tube?

Answer: ________________

c. If the radius of a tube, which has a driving pressure of 16 cm H_2O is reduced by 50% of its original size, what will be the new driving pressure required to maintain the same gas flow through the tube?

Answer: ________________

d. If the radius of a tube, which has a driving pressure of 10 cm H_2O, is reduced by 16% of its original size, what will be the new driving pressure required to maintain the same gas flow through the tube?

Answer ________________

e. If the radius of a tube, which has gas flowing through it at 50 liters per minute, is increased by 50% of its original size, what will be the new gas flow through the tube?

Answer ____________________

f. If the radius of a tube, which has gas flowing through it at 100 liters per minute, is increased by 16% of its original size, what will be the new gas flow through the tube?

Answer ____________________

g. If the radius of a tube, which has a driving pressure of 80 cm H_2O, is increased by 50% of its original size, what will be the new driving pressure required to maintain the same gas flow through the tube?

Answer ____________________

h. If the radius of a tube, which has a driving pressure of 5 cm H_2O, is increased by 16% of its original size, what will be the new driving pressure required to maintain the same gas flow through the tube?

Answer ____________________

6. Write the simple proportionalities of Poiseuille's Law for flow ($\dot{V}$) and pressure (P).

$\dot{V}$ =

P =

7. Airway resistance (R_{aw}) is defined as the: ________________________

____

____

8. Write the equation for airway resistance (R_{aw}) and include the units of measurement.

R_{aw} =

9. If a patient produces a flow rate of 10 L/second during inspiration by generating a transairway pressure of 30 cm H_2O, what is the patient's R_{aw}?

Answer ________________

SECTION D

1. The normal R_{aw} in the tracheobronchial tree is about ____________ to ______________ cm H_2O/L/sec.

2. Laminar gas flow refers to: ____________________________________

____

3. Turbulent gas flow refers to: ____________________________________

____

4. Time constant is defined as the: ____________________________________

____

____

____

5. Lung regions that have an increased airway resistance, require:

   a. Less time to inflate
   b. More time to inflate
   c. No change in time to inflate

6. Lung regions that have an increased compliance, require:

   a. Less time to inflate
   b. More time to inflate
   c. No change in time to inflate

7. Which of the following cause lung regions to have a long time constant?

   I. Decreased airway resistance
   II. Increased lung compliance
   III. Increased airway resistance
   IV. Decreased lung compliance

   a. I only
   b. III only
   c. II and III only
   d. III and IV only
   e. II, III, and IV only

8. Lung regions that have a decreased airway resistance, require:

   a. Less time to inflate
   b. More time to inflate
   c. No change in time to inflate

9. Lung regions that have a decreased compliance, require:

   a. Less time to inflate
   b. More time to inflate
   c. No change in time to inflate

10. Which of the following cause lung regions to have a short time constant?

    I. Increased airway resistance
    II. Decreased lung compliance
    III. Decreased airway resistance
    IV. Increased lung compliance

    a. II only
    b. IV only
    c. III only
    d. I and IV only
    e. II and III only

11. **Dynamic compliance** is defined as the: ____________________

    ____

    ____

    ____

12. In the normal lung, the dynamic compliance is (_____ equal to; _____ greater than; _____ less than) static compliance at all breathing frequencies.

13. In the partially obstructed airways, the ratio of dynamic compliance to static compliance (_____ increases; _____ decreases; _____ remains the same) as the breathing frequency increases.

14. **Frequency dependent** refers to: ____________________

    ____

    ____

    ____

    ____

SECTION E

1. The **ventilatory pattern** consists of the following three components:

   a.____

   b.____

   c.____

2. The normal tidal volume is about ___ to ___ml/kg; or ___to ___ml/lb.

3. The normal adult ventilatory rate is about ______ breaths per minute.

4. The normal I:E is about ____:____.

5. The gas that reaches the alveoli during inspiration is referred to as ______________________________.

6. The gas that does not reach the alveoli during inspiration is referred to as ______________________________.

7. Anatomic deadspace is defined as:______________________________

   ____

   ____

   ____

8. If a patient weighs 130 pounds, about how many milliliters (ml) of inspired gas during each breath would be anatomic deadspace gas?

   Answer ______________

9. **Alveolar ventilation** is equal to the ________________ minus the ______________________________ multiplied by the ______________________________.

10. If an individual presents this data:

- V_T = 575 ml
- V_D = 185 ml
- Breaths/minute = 16

what is the alveolar ventilation?

Answer ________________

11. **Alveolar deadspace** is defined as: ______________________________

____

____

12. **Physiologic deadspace** is defined as: __________________________

____

13. In the upright position, the negative intrapleural pressure at the apex of the lung is normally (_____ less; _____ greater) than at the base.

14. In the upright position, the alveoli in the upper lung regions are (_____ less; _____ greater; _____ equal) in size compared to the alveoli in the lower lung regions.

15. In the upright lung, ventilation is much greater in the:

a. Upper lung regions
b. Middle lung regions
c. Lower lung regions

16. When lung compliance decreases, the patient's ventilatory rate generally (_____ increases; _____ decreases; _____ remains the same) and the tidal volume (_____ increases; _____ decreases; _____ remains the same).

17. When airway resistance increases, the patient's ventilatory rate generally (_____ increases; _____ decreases; _____ remains the same) and the tidal volume (_____ increases; _____ decreases; _____ remains the same).

18. In response to a certain respiratory disorder, the patient may adopt a ventilatory pattern based on the expenditure of

_____________________________ rather than the efficiency of

______________________________________.

19. **Apnea** is defined as the: ______________________________________

____

20. **Eupnea** is defined as: ____

____

21. **Biot's Breathing** is defined as: ________________________________

____

____

____

22. **Hyperpnea** is defined as: ______________________________________

____

____

23. **Hyperventilation** is defined as: ________________________________

____

____

____

24. **Hypoventilation** is defined as: _________________________________

____

____

____

25. **Tachypnea** is defined as: ______________________________________

____

26. **Cheyne-Stokes** is defined as: ______________________________

____

____

____

____

____

27. **Kussmaul Breathing** is defined as: ______________________________

____

____

28. **Orthopnea** is defined as: ______________________________

____

____

____

29. **Dyspnea** is defined as: ______________________________

____

____

Chapter Three
The Diffusion of Pulmonary Gases

SECTION A

1. **Diffusion** is defined as: ____________________

____

____

____

____

2. **Boyle's Law** states that: ____________________

____

____

____

3. Boyle's Law is written as follows:

4. If an airtight container, which has a volume of 400 ml and a pressure of 50 cm H_2O, has its volume reduced to 300 ml, what will be the new pressure in the container?

Answer ____________________

5. If an airtight container, which has a volume of 55 ml and a pressure of 75 cm H_2O, has its volume increased to 110 ml, what will be the new pressure in the container?

Answer ______________________________

6. **Charles' Law** states that: ______________________________

____

____

____

7. Charles' Law is written as follows:

8. If the temperature of gas in an 8-liter balloon is increased from 290° Kelvin to 340° Kelvin, what will be the new volume in the balloon?

Answer ______________________________

9. If the temperature of an automobile tire, which has 4.5 liters of gas in it, is increased from 32° Celsius to 42° Celsius, what will be the new volume in the tire?

Answer ______________________________

10. **Gay-Lussac's Law** states that: ______________________________

____

____

____

11. Gay-Lussac's Law is written as follows:

12. If the temperature of the gas in a closed container, which has a pressure of 15 cm H_2O, is increased from 36° Kelvin to 375° Kelvin, what will be the new pressure in the container?

Answer______________________

13. If the temperature of the gas in a closed container, which has a pressure of 46 cm H_2O, is decreased from 40° Celsius to 30° Celsius, what will be the new pressure in the container?

Answer___________________

14. **Dalton's Law** states that: ______________________________________

____

____

____

15. The following gases and their respective pressures are enclosed in a container:

Gas	Partial Pressure
Nitrogen	470 mm Hg
Oxygen	130 mm Hg
Carbon Dioxide	50 mm Hg

According to Dalton's Law, what is the total pressure in the container?

Answer ___________________

SECTION B

1. At sea level, identify the percentage of the atmosphere and the partial pressure of the following gases that compose the barometric pressure:

TABLE 3–1. Gases that Compose the Barometric Pressure

GAS	% OF ATMOSPHERE	PARTIAL PRESSURE (mm Hg)
Nitrogen (N_2)		
Oxygen (O_2)		
Argon (Ar)		
Carbon Dioxide (CO_2)		

2. As one ascends a mountain, the barometric pressure (_____ increases; _____ decreases; _____ remains the same) and the percent concentration of oxygen (_____ increases; _____ decreases; _____ remains the same).

3. Compare and contrast the partial pressure of gases in the dry air, alveoli, arterial blood, and venous blood.

TABLE 3–2. Partial Pressure (in mm Hg) of Gases in the Air, Alveoli, and Blood*

GASES	DRY AIR	ALVEOLAR GAS	ARTERIAL BLOOD	VENOUS BLOOD
P_{O_2}				
P_{CO_2}				
P_{H_2O} (water vapor)				
P_{N_2} (and other gases in minute quantities)				
Total				

*The values shown are based upon standard pressure and temperature.

4. The reason the partial pressure of oxygen in the atmosphere is so much higher than the partial pressure of oxygen in the alveoli is because:

____

____

____

____

5. At body temperature, the alveolar gas has an absolute humidity of

____________ and a water vapor pressure (P_{H_2O}) of ______________.

6. If a patient is receiving an FI_{O_2} of .70 on a day when the barometric pressure is 748 mm Hg, and if the Pa_{CO_2} is 50 mm Hg, what is the patient's alveolar oxygen tension (PA_{O_2})?

Answer ________________

SECTION C

1. List the structures of the alveolar-capillary membrane that gas molecules must diffuse through the:

   a. ______________________________

   b. ______________________________

   c. ______________________________

   d. ______________________________

   e. ______________________________

   f. ______________________________

   g. ______________________________

   h. ______________________________

   i. ______________________________

2. The thickness of the alveolar-capillary membrane is between

______________ to ______________.

3. In the healthy resting person, the average $P\bar{v}_{O_2}$ is ______________ mm Hg and the average $P\bar{v}_{CO_2}$ is ________________ mm Hg.

4. Under normal circumstances, when venous blood enters the alveolar-capillary system, there is an oxygen pressure gradient of about ____________ mm Hg, and a carbon dioxide pressure gradient of about

____________ mm Hg.

5. The equilibrium of oxygen and carbon dioxide in the alveolar-capillary system is usually accomplished in about ______________ seconds.

6. The total transit time for blood to move through the alveolar-capillary system is about ___________ seconds, which is about

________________ of the time available.

7. During exercise, the time available for gas diffusion:

   a. increases
   b. decreases
   c. remains the same

8. **Fick's Law** is written as follows:

$$\dot{V} \text{ gas} =$$

9. According to Fick's Law, as the:

   I. Thickness decreases, gas diffusion:

      a. increases
      b. decreases
      c. remains the same

   II. Pressure difference increases, gas diffusion:

      a. increases
      b. decreases
      c. remains the same

   III. Area decreases, gas diffusion:

      a. increases
      b. decreases
      c. remains the same

10. **Henry's Law** states that: ____________________________________

____

____

____

11. The amount of gas that can be dissolved by 1 ml of a given liquid at standard pressure and specified temperature is known as the

____.

12. **Graham's Law** states that the rate of diffusion of a gas through

a liquid is (1)____

____

____

and (2) ____

____

____

13. **Perfusion Limited** means that: ______________________________

____

____

____

14. **Diffusion Limited** means that: ______________________________

____

____

____

15. Under normal circumstances, the diffusion of oxygen is:

   a. Perfusion limited
   b. Diffusion limited
   c. Neither perfusion nor diffusion limited

Chapter Four
Pulmonary Function Measurements

SECTION A

1. **Tidal Volume** (V_T) is defined as: ________________________________

____

____

2. **Inspiratory Reserve Volume** (IRV) is defined as: ________________

____

____

3. **Expiratory Reserve Volume** (ERV) is defined as: _________________

____

____

4. **Residual Volume** (RV) is defined as: ____________________________

____

____

5. **Vital Capacity** (VC) is defined as: _____________________________

____

____

6. **Inspiratory Capacity** (IC) is defined as: _______________________

____

____

7. **Functional Residual Capacity** (FRC) is defined as: ______________

____

____

8. **Total Lung Capacity** (TLC) is defined as: _______________________

____

____

9. **Residual Volume/Total Lung Capacity Ratio** (RV/TLC x 100) is defined as: ____

____

10. Compare and contrast the approximate lung volumes and capacities in the average normal male and female between 20 and 30 years of age.

TABLE 4–1. Approximate Lung Volumes and Capacities in the Average Normal Subject Between 20 and 30 Years of Age

	MALE		FEMALE	
MEASUREMENT	**ml**	**Approx. % of TLC**	**ml**	**Approx. % of TLC**
Tidal Volume (V_T)				
Inspiratory Reserve Volume (IRV)				
Expiratory Reserve Volume (ERV)				
Residual Volume (RV)				
Vital Capacity (VC)				
Inspiratory Capacity (IC)				
Functional Residual Capacity (FRC)				
Total Lung Capacity (TLC)		—		—
Residual Volume/Total Lung Capacity Ratio (RV/TLC × 100)				

11. In an obstructive lung disorder, the ____________, ____________, ________________, and ________________ are increased; and the ________, ________, ________, and ______________ are decreased.

12. In a restrictive lung disorder, the ____________, ____________, ____________, ____________, ____________, and ____________, are all decreased.

SECTION B

1. **Forced vital capacity** (FVC) is defined as:____________________

____

____

____

2. **Forced expiratory volume timed** (FEV_T) is defined as:__________

____

____

3. The normal percentage of the total volume exhaled during the following time periods are:

   a. $FEV_{0.5}$ _________%

   b. $FEV_{1.0}$ _________%

   c. $FEV_{2.0}$ _________%

   d. $FEV_{3.0}$ _________%

4. In obstructive disease, the percentage of FVC that can be forcefully exhaled over a specific period of time (___ decreases; ___ increases; ___ remains the same).

5. **Forced Expiratory Flow$_{200\text{-}1200}$** ($FEF_{200\text{-}1200}$) is defined as:

____

____

____

6. The $FEF_{200\text{-}1200}$ is a good index of the (___ large; ___ small) airway function.

7. **Forced Expiratory Flow$_{25\%\text{-}75\%}$** ($FEF_{25\%\text{-}75\%}$) is defined as:

____

____

____

8. The $FEF_{25\%-75\%}$ reflects the status of the ________________ to ___________ sized airways.

9. **Peak Expiratory Flow Rate** (PEFR) is defined as: ________________

____

____

10. **Maximum Voluntary Ventilation** (MVV) is defined as: _____________

____

____

11. **Forced Expiratory Volume$_1$ Second/Forced Vital Capacity Ratio** (FEV_1/FVC ratio) is defined as:

____

____

____

____

____

12. Label the following measurements graphically presented in the **flow-volume loop:**

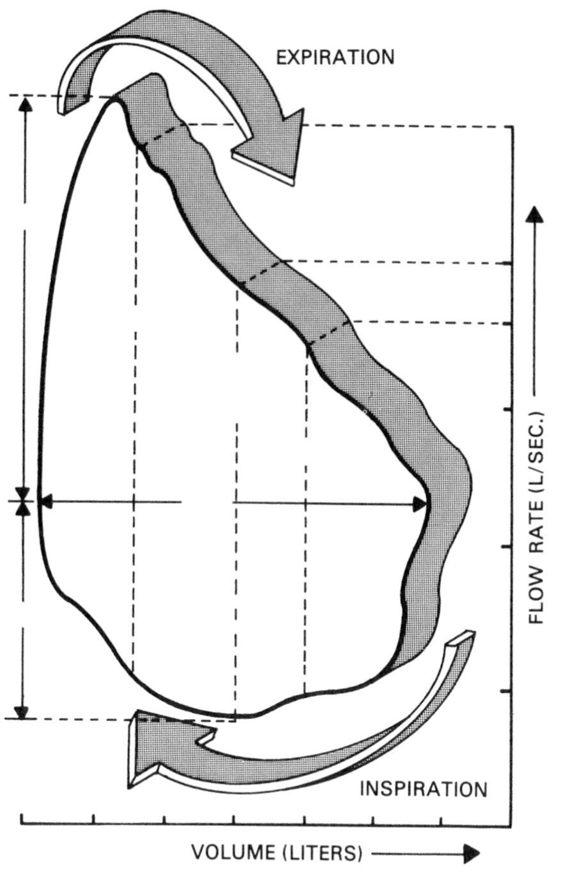

13. Compare and contrast the following average dynamic flow rate measurements of the healthy male and female between 20 and 30 years of age:

TABLE 4–2. Average Dynamic Flow Rate Measurements of the Healthy Male and Female Between 20 and 30 Years of Age

MEASUREMENT	MALE	FEMALE
FEV_T $FEV_{0.5}$ $FEV_{1.0}$ $FEV_{2.0}$ $FEV_{3.0}$		
$FEF_{200-1200}$		
$FEF_{25\%-75\%}$		
PEFR		
MVV		

14. Approximately the first 30% of a forced vital capacity maneuver is effort-dependent. **Effort-dependent** means that:

____

____

____

15. Approximately the last 70% of a forced vital capacity maneuver is effort-independent. **Effort-independent** means that:

____

____

____

16. The limitation of the flow rate that occurs during the last 70% of a forced vital capacity maneuver is due to the

____________________________________ of the walls of the airway.

17. As muscular effort and intrapleural pressure increase during a forced expiratory maneuver, the **equal pressure point** moves

____.

18. Once dynamic compression occurs during a forced expiratory maneuver, increased muscular effort (____ increases; ____ decreases; _____ has no effect on) airway compression.

CHAPTER FIVE
THE CIRCULATORY SYSTEM

SECTION A

1. List the four major components of blood.

   a. ______________________

   b ______________________

   c. ______________________

   d. ______________________

2. The ______________ constitute the major portion of the blood cells.

3. In the healthy adult male, there are about ________ million red blood cells in each cubic millimeter of blood.

4. In the healthy adult female, there are about ________ million red blood cells in each cubic millimeter of blood.

5. The percentage of red blood cells in relation to the total blood volume is known as the ______________.

6. Compare and contrast the normal hematocrit levels for the following:

   a. Adult male ________%

   b. Adult female ________%

   c. Newborn _____ to _____%

7. Microscopically, the red blood cells appear as biconcave disks, averaging about ________ in diameter and ________ in thickness.

8. The life span of a RBC is about ________ days.

9. The major function of the leukocytes is to:

   ____

   ____

   ____

   ____

10. The normal amount of leukocytes average between ________ to ________ cells per cubic millimeter of blood.

11. Compare and contrast the normal differential count for the following:

TABLE 5–1. Normal Differential Count

POLYMORPHONUCLEAR GRANULOCYTES	MONONUCLEAR CELLS
Neutrophils	Lymphocytes
Eosinophils	Monocytes
Basophils	

12. The most active leukocytes in response to tissue destruction by bacteria are the ________________________.

13. ________________________ are commonly elevated in response to an allergic condition.

14. ________________________ are commonly elevated in response to a chronic infection.

15. The ________________________ are involved in the production of antibodies.

16. Thrombocytes are also called ________________________.

17. The normal platelet count in each cubic millimeter of blood ranges between ________________________ and ________________________.

18. The function of the platelet is to: ________________________

____

____

____

19. Plasma constitutes about ______________ percent of the total blood volume.

20. Approximately ______________ percent of the plasma consists of water.

21. **Proteins** found in the plasma are:

a. ______________________________

b. ______________________________

c. ______________________________

22. **Electrolyte cations** found in the plasma are:

a. ______________________________

b. ______________________________

c. ______________________________

d. ______________________________

23. **Electrolyte anions** found in the plasma are:

a. ______________________________

b. ______________________________

c. ______________________________

d. ______________________________

24. **Food substances** found in the plasma are:

a. ______________________________

b. ______________________________

c. ______________________________

d. ______________________________

25. **Waste products** found in the plasma are:

a. ______________________________

b. ______________________________

c. ______________________________

d. ______________________________

SECTION B

1. Label and color the following anatomic structures of the heart:

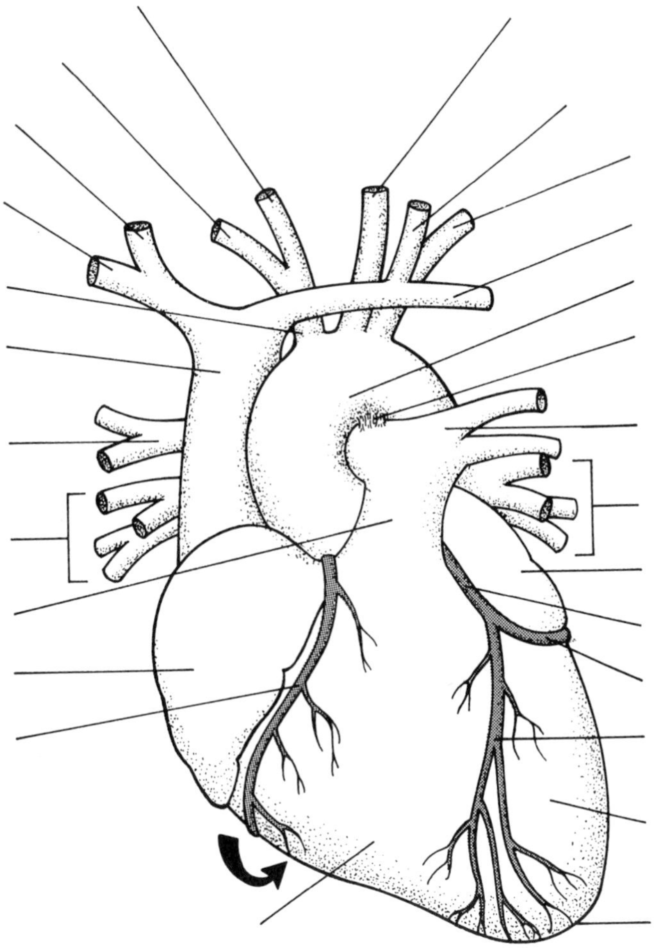

Anterior view of the heart.

2. The right atrium of the heart receives blood from the ____.

3. A one-way valve called the ____________________ lies between the right atrium and right ventricle.

4. The chordae tendineae are secured to the ventricular wall by the ______________________________.

5. Blood leaves the right ventricle through the ____________________ ____________________ and enters the right and left ________________ ________________________.

6. After blood passes through the lungs, it returns to the left atrium by way of the ____.

7. The bicuspid valve, which lies between the left atrium and left ventricle, is also called the ______________________________.

8. The left ventricle pumps blood through the ascending ________________________.

9. The __________________________________ valve prevents the backflow of blood into the left ventricle.

10. Using the following illustration, label the components of the conductive system of the heart:

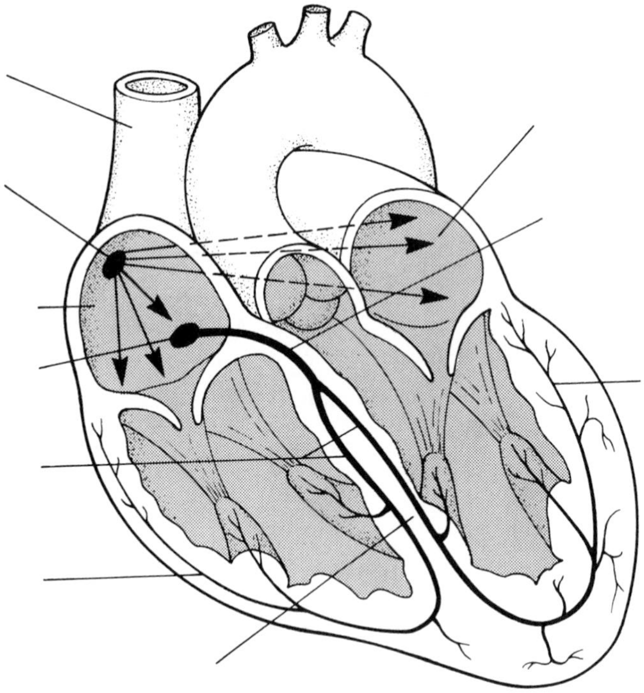

11. The pacemaker of the heart is the ____________________________.

12. The **cardioaccelerator center** increases heart rate and strength of contraction, by sending ____________________ impulse to the heart.

13. The **cardioinhibitor center** decrease the heart rate and strength of contraction by sending ____________________ impulses to the heart.

14. The **P wave** represents the ______________________________ ______________________________.

15. The **QRS complex** represents ______________________________ ______________________________.

16. The **T wave** represents ______________________________ ______________________________.

17. Identify the following components of a normal electrocardiogram:

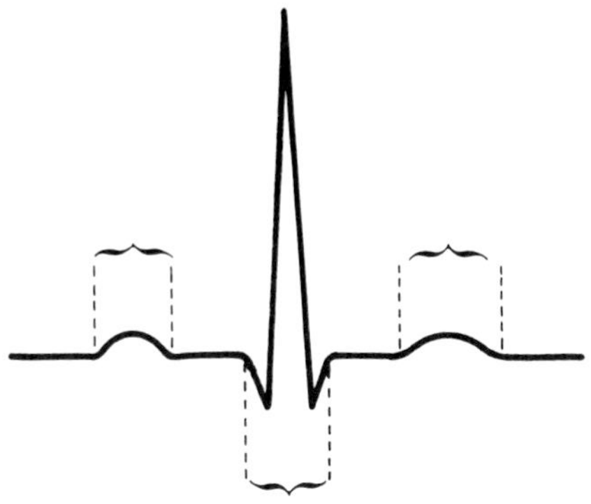

SECTION C

1. The normal adult heart rate is ____________________.

2. The normal infant heart rate is about ____________________.

3. The pulmonary circulation system begins with the ____________________ ____________________ and ends in the ____________________.

4. The system circulation system begins with the ____________________ and ends in the ____________________.

5. The arteries are vessels that carry blood (_____ to; _____ away from) the heart.

6. The arteries subdivide into smaller vessels called ____________________.

7. The ________________________ play a major role in the distribution and regulation of blood pressure.

8. What vessels are referred to as the resistance vessels?

Answer ____.

9. In the capillaries of the pulmonary system, gas exchange is called ______________________________ respiration.

10. In the capillaries of the systemic system, gas exchange is called ____________________________ respirations.

11. Tiny vessels continuous with the capillaries are called ____________________________.

12. Veins are also known as ______________________ vessels.

13. Approximately _____% of the body's total blood volume is contained within the venous system.

14. The pulmonary arterioles and most of the arterioles in the systemic circulation are controlled by _______________________ impulses.

15. The ____________________________________ center, located in the ______________________________, governs the number of__________________ impulses sent to the vascular systems.

16. Under normal circumstances, a continual stream of _________________________ impulses are sent to blood vessels.

17. A moderate state of constant vascular constriction is called ____.

18. When the vasomotor center is activated to constrict a particular vascular region, it does so by (_____ increasing; _____ decreasing) the number of ___________________ impulses sent to that vascular area.

19. When the vasomotor center causes vasodilation, it does so by (____ increasing; ____ decreasing) the number of ___________________ impulses sent to that vascular region.

20. List the major vascular beds in the systemic system that dilate in response to sympathetic impulses.

The arterioles of the :

a. ______________________________

b. ______________________________

c. ______________________________

21. **Baroreceptors**, which are specialized stretch receptors, are also called ______________________________.

22. The baroreceptors located in the carotid arteries send neural impulses to the medulla by means of the ______________________ nerve.

23. The baroreceptors located in the arch of the aorta send neural impulses to the medulla by means of the ______________ nerve.

24. When the arterial blood pressure decreases, neural impulses to the medulla (_____ increase; _____ decrease); which, in turn, causes the medulla to (_____ increase; _____ decrease) its sympathetic activity.

25. When the baroreceptors signal the medulla to increase its sympathetic activity, the net result is:

a. ____

____

b. ____

____

c. ____

____

26. In addition to the baroreceptors located in the carotid sinuses and aortic arch, other baroreceptors are found in the:

a. ______________________________

b. ______________________________

c. ______________________________

d. ______________________________

SECTION D

1. **Intravascular pressure** is defined as the: ____________________

____

____

____

2. **Transmural pressure** is defined as the: ____________________

____

____

____

3. A positive transmural pressure is when pressure inside the vessel is (____ greater than; ______ less than; _____ the same as) the pressure outside the vessel.

4. A negative transmural pressure is when the pressure inside the vessel is (____ greater than; ______ less than; _____ the same as) the pressure outside the vessel.

5. **Driving pressure** is defined as the: ____________________

____

____

____

6. The maximum pressure generated during ventricular contraction is the ______________________________________.

7. When the ventricles relax, the lowest pressure that remains in the arteries prior to the next ventricular contraction is the

____.

8. Compared to the pulmonary circulation, the pressure in the systemic system is about _________ times greater.

9. Using the illustration below, identify the following mean intraluminal blood pressures at various points in the pulmonary and systemic circulation:

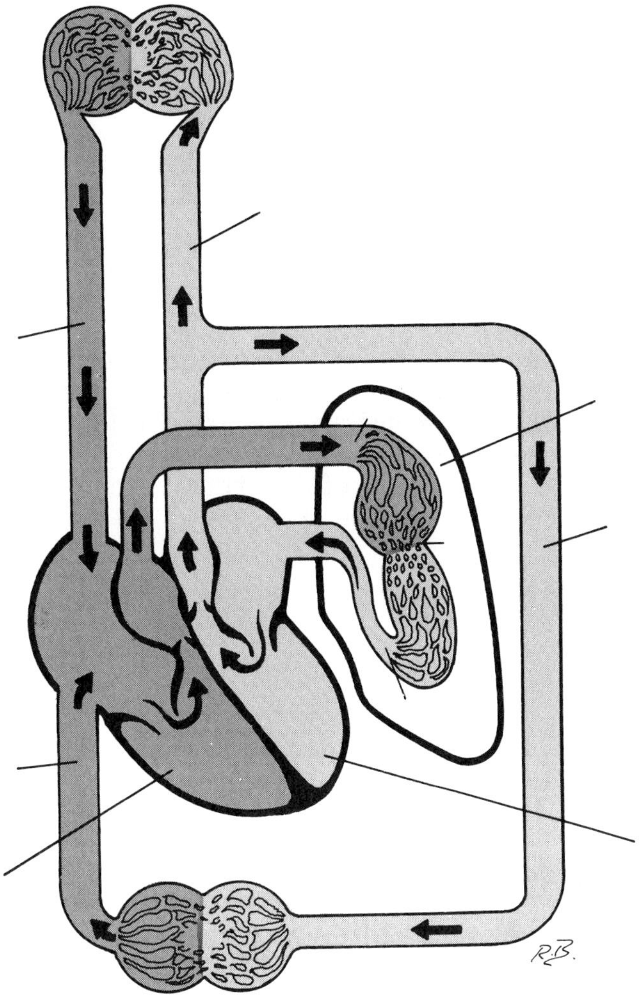

10. Normally, the stroke volume ranges between ______________ and ___________________.

11. The total volume of blood discharged from the ventricles per minute is called ____.

12. If an individual has a stroke volume of 55 ml, and a heart rate of 80 beats per minute, what is the cardiac output?

ANSWER ______________________________

13. Under normal conditions, when either the stroke volume or heart rate increases, the blood pressure:

    a. Increases
    b. Decreases
    c. Remains the same

14. The normal adult total blood volume is about __________ liters.

15. In regard to the total blood volume of the normal adults, about _____ percent is in the systemic circulation, _____ percent is in the heart, and _____ percent is in the pulmonary circulation.

16. Overall, about _____ percent of the total blood volume is in the veins, and about _____ percent is in the arteries.

SECTION E

1. The fact that blood is **gravity-dependent** means that it naturally

   moves: ____

   ____

   ____

2. The intraluminal pressures in the vessels of the gravity-dependent areas of the lung are (____ greater than; ____ less than; ____ the same as) the intraluminal pressures in the least gravity-dependent areas.

3. When an individual is in the following position, what part of the lung is the gravity-dependent region?

Body Position	Gravity-Dependent Lung Region
a. Lying on the back	____________________
b. Lying on the stomach	____________________
c. Lying on the side	____________________
d. Suspended upside down	____________________

4. In **zone 1** of the upright lung, the alveolar pressure is sometimes (____ greater than; ____ less than; ____ the same as) both the arterial and the venous intraluminal pressures.

5. List some conditions that can cause the alveolar pressure to be higher than the arterial and venous pressures.

   a. ____

   b. ____

   c. ____

6. When the alveoli are ventilated but not perfused, ______________

   ____________________________ is said to exist.

7. In **zone 2** of the upright lung, the arterial intraluminal pressure is (____ greater than; ____ less than; ____ the same as) the alveolar pressure; and the alveolar pressure is (____ greater than; ____ less than; ____ the same as) the venous pressure.

8. In **zone 3** of the upright lung, the arterial intraluminal pressure is (____ greater than; ____ less than; ____ the same as) the alveolar pressure; and the alveolar pressure is (____ greater than; ____ less than; ____ the same as) the venous pressure.

9. List the three mechanisms that determine stroke volume.

   a. ____

   b. ____

   c. ____

10. **Ventricular preload** refers to: ____________________________

    ____

    ____

11. Within limits, the more myocardial fiber is stretched during diastole, the (____ more; ____ less) strongly it will contract during systole.

12. **VEDP** stands for: ____________________________

13. **VEDV** stands for: ____________________________

14. As the VEDV increase the VEDP:

    a. increase
    b. decrease
    c. remains the same

15. The relationship between the VEDP and cardiac output is known as the: ____.

16. **Ventricular afterload** is defined as: ______________________________

____

____.

17. Ventricular afterload is determined by:

a. ____

____

b. ____

____

c. ____

____

18. Clinically, what reflects the ventricular afterload the best?

Answer: ____

19. **Blood pressure** (BP) equals:

BP = ______________ x _______________

20. **Myocardial contractility** can be pictured as: ____________________

____

____

____

21. In general, when the contractility of the heart decreases, the cardiac output:

a. increases
b. decreases
c. remains the same

22. List some clinical assessments that reflect myocardial contractility.

    a. ______________________________

    b. ______________________________

    c. ______________________________

    d. ______________________________

23. An increase in myocardial contractility is referred to as __________

    ______________________________.

24. A decrease in myocardial contractility is referred to as __________

    ______________________________.

25. Circulatory resistance is derived as follows:

    Resistance =

26. In general, when the vascular resistance increases, the blood pressure:

    a. increases
    b. decreases
    c. remains the same

SECTION F

1. Define **active mechanism.** ______________________________

   ____

   ____

   ____

2. In response to a decreased alveolar oxygen pressure, the pulmonary vascular system:

   a. constricts
   b. relaxes
   c. remains the same

3. In response to an increased P_{CO_2} level, the pulmonary vascular system:

   a. constricts
   b. relaxes
   c. remains the same

4. In response to a decreased pH, the pulmonary vascular system:

   a. constricts
   b. relaxes
   c. remains the same

5. In response to an increase H^+ concentration, the pulmonary vascular system:

   a. constricts
   b. relaxes
   c. remains the same

6. List some pharmacologic agents that constrict the pulmonary vascular.

   a. ______________________________
   b. ______________________________
   c. ______________________________
   d. ______________________________
   e. ______________________________

7. List some pharmacologic agents that relax the pulmonary vascular.

   a. ______________________________
   b. ______________________________
   c. ______________________________
   d. ______________________________

8. List some pathologic conditions that increase pulmonary vascular resistance.

   a. ______________________________
   b. ______________________________

SECTION G

1. Define **passive mechanism.** ____

____

____

____

2. In response to an increased pulmonary arterial pressure, the pulmonary vascular resistance:

   a. increases
   b. decreases
   c. remains the same

3. The answer to the above question occurs because of recruitment,

   which entails ____

   ____

   and because of distention, which entails ____________________

   ____

   ____

4. In response to an increased left atrial pressure, the pulmonary vascular resistance:

   a. increases
   b. decreases
   c. remains the same

5. At high lung volumes, the pulmonary resistance in the alveolar vessels is (____ high; ____ low).

6. At high lung volumes, the pulmonary resistance in the extra-alveloar vessels is: (____ high; ____ low).

7. At low lung volumes, the pulmonary resistance in the alveolar vessels is (____ high; ____ low).

8. At low lung volumes, the pulmonary resistance in the extra-alveolar vessels is: (____ high; ____ low).

9. At high lung volumes, the pulmonary vascular resistance in the corner vessels is: (____ high; ____ low).

10. At low lung volumes, the pulmonary vascular resistance in the corner vessels is (____ high; ____ low).

11. In response to an increased blood volume, pulmonary vascular resistance:

    a. increases
    b. decreases
    c. remains the same

12. In response to an increased blood viscosity, the pulmonary vascular resistance:

    a. increases
    b. decreases
    c. remains the same

CHAPTER SIX
HEMODYNAMIC MEASUREMENTS

SECTION A

1. **Hemodynamic** is defined as:______________________________

____

____

2. Write the abbreviation and normal range for the following hemodynamic values directly obtained by means of the pulmonary artery catheter:

TABLE 6–1. Hemodynamic Values Directly Obtained by Means of the Pulmonary Artery Catheter

HEMODYNAMIC VALUE	ABBREVIATION	NORMAL RANGE
Central venous pressure		
Right atrial pressure		
Mean pulmonary artery pressure		
Pulmonary capillary wedge pressure (also called pulmonary artery wedge; pulmonary artery occlusion)		
Cardiac output		

3. Write the abbreviation and normal range for the following computed hemodynamic values:

TABLE 6–2. Computed Hemodynamic Values

HEMODYNAMIC VARIABLE	ABBREVIATION	NORMAL RANGE
Stroke volume		
Stroke volume index		
Cardiac index		
Right ventricular stroke work index		
Left ventricular stroke work index		
Pulmonary vascular resistance		
Systemic vascular resistance		

SECTION B

1. **Stroke volume** (SV) is defined as:____________________________

____

____

2. List the major determinants of stroke volume.

a.____

b.____

c.____

3. Complete the following equation:

SV =

4. If a patient has a cardiac output of 5.5 L/min and a heart rate of 87 beats/min., what is the stroke volume?

Answer:________________

5. The **stroke volume index** (SVI) is derived by:____________________

____

____

6. If a patient has a stroke volume of 55 ml and a body surface area of 2.5 m^2, what is the SVI?

Answer:________________

7. Clinically, what does the SVI reflect?

a.____

b.____

c.____

8. The **cardiac index** (CI) is calculated by:________________________

____

____

9. If a patient has a cardiac output of 7 L/min and a body surface area of 2.5 m^2, what is the CI?

Answer:________________

10. What does the **right ventricular stroke work index** (RVSWI) measure?

Answer:____

____

____

11. Clinically, what does the RVSWI reflect?

Answer:____

____

12. Complete the following equation:

RVSWI =

13. If a patient has a SVI of 40 ml, a $\overline{PA}$ of 25 mm Hg, and a CVP of 10 mm Hg, what is the RVSWI?

Answer:________________________

14. What does the **left ventricular stroke work index** (LVSWI) measure?

Answer:____

____

____

15. Clinically, what does the LVSWI reflect?

Answer:____

____

16. Complete the following equation:

LVSWI =

17. If a patient has a SVI of 45 ml, an MAP of 125 mm Hg, and a PCWP of 10 mm Hg, what is the LVSWI?

Answer:__________________

18. List factors that increase and decrease the following:

TABLE 6–3. Factors Increasing and Decreasing Stroke Volume (SV), Stroke Volume Index (SVI), Cardiac Output (CO), Cardiac Index (CI), Right Ventricular Stroke Work Index (RVSWI), and Left Ventricular Stroke Work Index (LVSWI)

INCREASES	DECREASES
Drugs (Increased Contractility)	**Drugs (Decreased Contractility)**
	Abnormal Conditions
Abnormal Conditions	
	Hyperinflation of Lungs

19. The pulmonary vascular system is a (____ high; ____ low) resistance system.

20. The systemic vascular system is a (____ high; ____ low) resistance system.

21. Clinically, what does **pulmonary vascular resistance** (PVR) indicate?

Answer:____

22. Complete the following equation:

PVR =

23. If a patient has a $\overline{PA}$ of 20, a PCWP of 10 mm Hg, and a CO of 7 L/min, what is the PVR?

Answer:________________________

24. List factors under the following categories that increase pulmonary vascular resistance:

TABLE 6–4. Factors that Increase Pulmonary Vascular Resistance (PVR)

CHEMICAL STIMULI	**PATHOLOGIC FACTORS**
PHARMACOLOGIC AGENTS	
HYPERINFLATION OF LUNGS	
	HUMORAL SUBSTANCES

25. List factors under the following categories that decrease pulmonary vascular resistance:

TABLE 6–5. Factors that Decrease Pulmonary Vascular Resistance (PVR)

PHARMACOLOGIC AGENTS	HUMORAL SUBSTANCES

26. Clinically, what does **systemic vascular resistance** (SVR) indicate?

Answer:____

27. Complete the following equation:

SVR =

28. If a patient has a MAP of 105 mm Hg, a CVP of 10 mm Hg, and a CO of 6 L/min, what is the SVR?

Answer:____________________________

29. List factors under the following category that increase and decrease the SVR:

TABLE 6–6. Factors that Increase and Decrease Systemic Vascular Resistance (SVR)

INCREASES	DECREASES
Vasoconstricting Agents	**Vasodilating Agents**
Abnormal Conditions	
	Abnormal Conditions

CHAPTER SEVEN
OXYGEN TRANSPORT

SECTION A

1. Compare and contrast the normal blood gas value ranges for the following:

	Normal Blood Gas Ranges	
Blood Gas	Arterial	Venous
pH		
P_{CO_2}		
HCO_3^-		
P_{O_2}		

2. The term **"dissolved"** means that when a gas like oxygen enters the plasma, it ______________________________

____

____

____

3. Clinically, what portion of the oxygen transport system is measured to assess the patient's partial pressure of oxygen (PO_2)?

ANSWER: ______________________________

4. Complete the following exercise.

PART I:

If an individual has an arterial oxygen partial pressure (Pa_{O_2}) of 50 mm Hg, about how many ml of oxygen is dissolved in every 100 ml of blood?

ANSWER: ____________ ml O_2/100 ml of blood.

PART II:

In regard to the above answer, what is the vol% of dissolved oxygen?

ANSWER: ________________

5. Vol% (volumes percent) is defined as: __________________________

____

6. Each red blood cell (RBC) contains approximately ________ million hemoglobin molecules.

7. The normal adult hemoglobin is designated as Hb __________.

8. In the normal adult hemoglobin, how many heme group(s) are there?

ANSWER ______________________________________

9. Write the reversible reaction of O_2 with Hb.

10. When two oxygen molecules are bound to one Hb molecule, the Hb is said to be _____% saturated with oxygen; a Hb molecule with one oxygen molecule is _____% saturated.

11. Hemoglobin bound with oxygen is called ______________________________.

12. Hemoglobin not bound with oxygen is called _____________________________ or ______________________________.

13. The amount of oxygen bound to hemoglobin is (_______ indirectly; _______ directly) related to the partial pressure of oxygen.

14. The **globin portion** of each hemoglobin molecule consists of:

____

____

____

15. **Fetal hemoglobin** (HbF) has __________ chains and __________ chains.

16. Hemoglobin changed from the ferrous state to the ferric state is known as ____________________________.

17. Compare and contrast the normal hemoglobin values for the following:

    a. Adult male ________ g% Hb

    b. Adult female _______ g% Hb

    c. Average infant _____ g% Hb

18. Hemoglobin constitutes about _____% of the RBC weight.

19. Each g% Hb is capable of carrying about _______ ml of oxygen.

20. At a normal arterial oxygen pressure (Pa_{O_2}) the hemoglobin saturation (Sa_{O_2}) is only 97% because of the following normal physiologic shunts:

    a. ____

    ____

    b. ____

    ____

    c. ____

    ____

SECTION B

1. Complete the following total oxygen transport exercises:

CASE A

A 23-year-old female with severe asthma presents the following clinical data:

Hb: 13 g%

Pa_{O_2}: 55 mm Hg

Sa_{O_2}: 85%

Cardiac Output: 6 L/minute

QUESTION 1. How much dissolved O_2 is the patient transporting in every 100 ml of blood?

ANSWER______________________ ml O_2/100 ml blood (vol%)

QUESTION 2. How much O_2 is bound to the hemoglobin in every 100 ml of blood?

ANSWER______________________________ ml O_2/100 ml blood (vol%)

QUESTION 3. What is the total O_2 content of the arterial blood (Ca_{O_2})?

ANSWER: Ca_{O_2} = ____________________ (Vol% O_2; or ml O_2/100 ml blood)

QUESTION 4. Since the Ca_{O_2} is in reference to 1/10 of one liter of blood, how many ml of O_2 are available for tissue metabolism in one liter of blood?

ANSWER________________________ml O_2/liter

QUESTION 5. Since this patient has a cardiac output of 6 liters/minute, how many ml of O_2 are available for tissue metabolism in one minute?

ANSWER____________________ml O_2/minute

CASE B

A 62-year-old male with severe emphysema presents the following clinical data:

- Hb: 18 g%
- Pa_{O_2}: 50 mm Hg
- Sa_{O_2}: 80%
- Cardiac Output: 3.5 L/minute
- $P\bar{v}_{O_2}$: 25 mm Hg
- $S\bar{v}_{O_2}$: 50%
- PA_{O_2}: 150 mm Hg

QUESTION 1. How much dissolved O_2 is the patient transporting in every 100 ml of blood?

ANSWER________________ml O_2/100 ml blood (vol%)

QUESTION 2. How much O_2 is bound to the hemoglobin in every 100 ml of blood?

ANSWER________________ml O_2/100 ml blood (vol% O)

QUESTION 3. What is the total O_2 content of the arterial blood (Ca_{O_2})?

ANSWER: Ca_{O_2} = ______________ (vol% O_2; or ml O_2/100 ml blood)

QUESTION 4. Since the Ca_{O_2} is in reference to 1/10 of one liter of blood, how many ml of O_2 are available for tissue metabolism in one liter of blood?

ANSWER: ________________ ml O_2/liter

QUESTION 5. Since this patient has a cardiac output of 3.5 liters/minute, how many ml of O_2 are available for tissue metabolism in one minute?

ANSWER: ________________ ml O_2/minute

QUESTION 6. What is the patient's total oxygen content of mixed venous blood ($C\bar{v}_{O_2}$)?

ANSWER: $C\bar{v}_{O_2}$ = ________________ (vol% O_2; or ml O_2/100 ml blood)

QUESTION 7. What is the patient's total oxygen content of capillary blood (Cc_{O_2})?

ANSWER: Cc_{O_2} = ________________ (vol% O_2; or ml O_2/100 ml blood)

SECTION C

1. The **oxygen dissociation curve** illustrates the__________________ of hemoglobin that is chemically bound to oxygen at each oxygen ______________________.

2. Clinically, the **flat portion** of the oxygen dissociation curve is significant because it illustrates that:

   a. ____

   ____

   ____

   b. ____

   ____

   ____

   c. ____

   ____

   ____

3. Clinically, the **steep portion** of the oxygen dissociation curve is significant because it illustrates that:

   a. ____

   ____

   ____

   b. ____

   ____

4. Using the following oxygen dissociation curve nomogram, answer questions a and b.

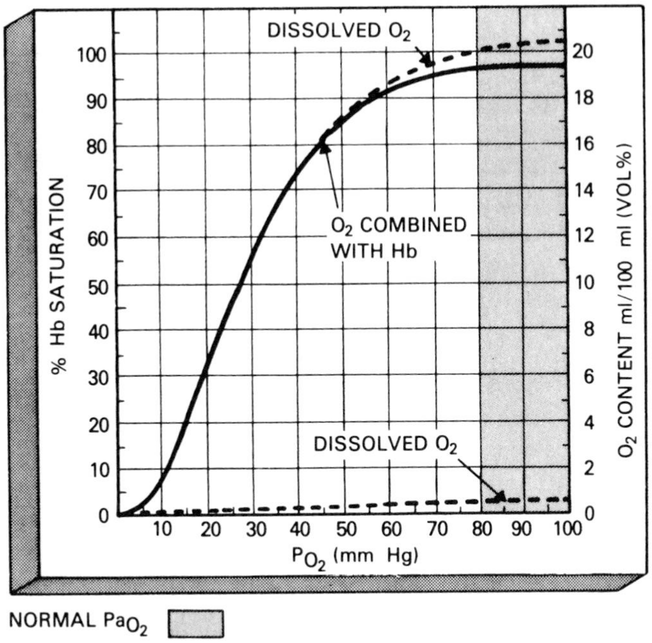

Oxygen dissociation curve

a. If the P_{O_2} is 50 mm Hg, what is the percentage of hemoglobin that is bound to oxygen?

ANSWER____________________________

b. What is the oxygen content level in vol%?

ANSWER____________________________

5. The $\mathbf{P_{50}}$ represents:____

____

____

6. Normally, the P_{50} is about ___________mm Hg.

7. When the oxygen dissociation curve shifts to the right, the P_{50}:

a. increases
b. decreases
c. remains the same

8. When the oxygen dissociation curve shifts to the left, the P_{50}:

a. increases
b. decreases
c. remains the same

9. List factors that shift the oxygen dissociation curve to the:

   a. Left: ______________________

   ____

   ____

   ____

   ____

   ____

   b. Right: ______________________

   ____

   ____

   ____

10. Clinically, when the oxygen dissociation curve shifts to the <u>right</u>, the loading of oxygen in the lungs at any given P_{O_2}:

    a. increases
    b. decreases
    c. remains the same

11. Clinically, when the oxygen dissociation curve shifts to the <u>right</u>, the plasma P_{O_2} reduction necessary to unload oxygen at the tissue sites is:

    a. less than normal
    b. greater than normal
    c. the same as normal

12. Clinically, when the oxygen dissociation curve shifts to the <u>left</u>, the loading of oxygen in the lungs at any given P_{O_2}:

    a. increases
    b. decreases
    c. remains the same

13. Clinically, when the oxygen dissociation curve shifts to the <u>left</u>, the plasma P_{O_2} reduction necessary to unload oxygen at the tissue sites is:

    a. less than normal
    b. greater than normal
    c. the same as normal

SECTION D

1. List the most common oxygen transport studies performed in the clinical setting.

   a. ______________________________

   b. ______________________________

   c. ______________________________

   d. ______________________________

   e. ______________________________

   f. ______________________________

2. **Total oxygen delivery** to the peripheral tissues is dependent on the:

   a. ______________________________

   b. ______________________________

   c. ______________________________

3. Complete the following formula:

$$\dot{D}_{O_2} =$$

4. If a patient has a cardiac output of 3.5 L/minute and an Ca_{O_2} of 12 vol%, what is the total amount of oxygen delivered to the patient's peripheral cells?

ANSWER ______________________

5. List three conditions that reduce an individual's total oxygen delivery:

a. ______________________

b. ______________________

c. ______________________

6. The **arterial-venous content difference** [$C(a-\bar{v})_{O_2}$] is defined as

the difference: ______________________

____

7. Complete the following formula:

$C(a-\bar{v})_{O_2}$ =

8. If a patient has an Ca_{O_2} of 13 vol% and a $C\bar{v}_{O_2}$ of 9 vol%, what is the patient's $C(a-\bar{v})_{O_2}$?

ANSWER ____________________

9. List some clinical factors that <u>increase</u> the $C(a-\bar{v})_{O_2}$:

a. ____________________

b. ____________________

1) ____________________

2) ____________________

3) ____________________

4) ____________________

10. List some clinical factors that <u>decrease</u> the $C(a-\bar{v})_{O_2}$:

a. ____________________

b. ____________________

c. ____________________

d. ____________________

e. ____________________

11. The amount of oxygen extracted by the peripheral tissues during the period of one minute is called ______________________________ or ______________________________.

12. Complete the following formula:

$$\dot{V}_{O_2} =$$

13. If a patient has a cardiac output of 7.5 L/minute and an $C(a-\bar{v})_{O_2}$ of 8 vol%, what is the patient's $\dot{V}_{O_2}$?

ANSWER ____________________

14. List some clinical factors that <u>increase</u> the $\dot{V}_{O_2}$.

a. ______________________________

b. ______________________________

c. ______________________________

d. ______________________________

15. List some clinical factors that <u>decrease</u> the $\dot{V}_{O_2}$.

a. ____________________

b. ____________________

c. ____________________

d. ____________________

16. An individual's oxygen consumption index is derived by dividing the $\dot{V}_{O_2}$ by the ____________________.

17. The average oxygen consumption index ranges between __________ to __________ ml O_2/m^2.

18. The oxygen extraction ratio (O_2ER) is defined as the amount of oxygen:

____

____

____

____

19. The O_2ER is also known as the:

a. ____________________

b. ____________________

20. Complete the following formula:

O_2ER =

21. The normal O_2ER is __________%

22. PART I

If a patient has a Ca_{O_2} as 14 vol%, and a $C\bar{v}_{O_2}$ of 7 vol%, what is the patient's O_2ER.

ANSWER ____________________%

PART II

If the above patient has a total oxygen delivery of 850 ml/minute, then this would mean that during a course of one minute, __________ ml of oxygen are metabolized by the tissues and __________ ml of oxygen are returned to the lungs.

23. List some clinical factors that <u>increase</u> the O_2ER.

a. ______________________________

b. ______________________________

   1. ______________________________
   2. ______________________________
   3. ______________________________
   4. ______________________________

c. ______________________________

d. ______________________________

24. List some clinical factors that <u>decrease</u> the O_2ER.

a. ______________________________

b. ______________________________

c. ______________________________

d. ______________________________

e. ______________________________

f. ______________________________

25. The normal $S\bar{v}_{O_2}$ is ________ %.

26. Clinically, an $S\bar{v}_{O_2}$ of about ______% is acceptable.

27. List some clinical factors that <u>decrease</u> the $S\bar{v}_{O_2}$.

a. ______________________________

b. ______________________________

1. ______________________________

2. ______________________________

3. ______________________________

4. ______________________________

28. A reduction in the $S\bar{v}_{O_2}$ indicates that the $C(a-\bar{v})_{O_2}$, $\dot{V}_{O_2}$, and O_2ER are:

a. increasing
b. decreasing
c. remaining the same

29. List some clinical factors that <u>increase</u> the $S\bar{v}_{O_2}$.

a. ______________________________

b. ______________________________

c. ______________________________

d. ______________________________

e. ______________________________

30. An increase in the $S\bar{v}_{O_2}$ indicates that the $C(a-\bar{v})_{O_2}$, $\dot{V}_{O_2}$, and O_2ER are:

a. increasing
b. decreasing
c. remaining the same

31. Directions: Indicate with the following code system how the listed clinical factors will likely alter a patient's total oxygen delivery, $\dot{V}_{O_2}$, $C(a-\bar{v})_{O_2}$, O_2ER, and $S\bar{v}_{O_2}$.

Code System: Same = unchanged status; ↑ = increase; ↓ = decrease

TABLE 7–10. Clinical Factors Affecting Various Oxygen Transport Study Values

CLINICAL FACTORS	OXYGEN TRANSPORT STUDIES				
	D_{O_2} (1000 ml O_2/min)	$\dot{V}_{O_2}$ (250 ml O_2/min)	$C(a-\bar{v})_{O_2}$ (5 vol%)	O_2ER (25%)	$S\bar{v}_{O_2}$ (75%)
↑O_2 Consumption					
↓O_2 Consumption					
↓Cardiac Output					
↑Cardiac Output					
↓Pa_{O_2}					
↑Pa_{O_2}					
↓Hb					
↑Hb					
Peripheral Shunting					

↑: increase; ↓: decrease.

SECTION E

1. **Pulmonary shunting** is defined as: ______________________________

   ____
   ____
   ____
   ____
   ____
   ____
   ____
   ____

2. List the two major conditions that cause a true **shunt mechanism.**

   a. ____

   b. ____

3. An **anatomic shunt** exists when: ______________________________

   ____
   ____
   ____

4. The normal anatomic shunt is about __________ to __________%.

5. List three common causes of **anatomic shunting.**

   a. ____

   b. ____

   c. ____

6. List three common causes of **capillary shunting.**

   a. ____

   b. ____

   c. ____

7. The sum of the anatomic and capillary shunts is referred to as

   __________ or ______________________________.

8. What does **refractory** to oxygen therapy mean?

____

____

____

____

____

____

9. A **shunt-like effect** is said to exist when: ______________________

____

____

10. List some common causes of the shunt-like effect mechanism.

a. ____

b. ____

c. ____

11. What is **venous admixture**?

____

____

____

12. Complete the following shunt equation:

$$\frac{\dot{Q}s}{\dot{Q}t} =$$

13. Case Study: Pneumonia Patient

A 42-year-old female is on a volume-cycled mechanical ventilator on a day when the barometric pressure is 740 mm Hg. The patient is receiving an FI_{O_2} of .45. The following clinical data are obtained:

Hb: 10 g%

Pa_{O_2}: 65 mm Hg (Sa_{O_2} = 91%)

Pa_{CO_2}: 35 mm Hg

$P\bar{v}_{O_2}$: 30 mm Hg ($S\bar{v}_{O_2}$ = 60%)

With the above information, calculate the patient's PA_{O_2}, Cc_{O_2}, Ca_{O_2}, and $C\bar{v}_{O_2}$.

a. PA_{O_2} =

Answer: ____________________

b. Cc_{O_2} =

Answer: ____________________

c. Ca_{O_2} =

Answer: ____________________

d. $C\bar{v}_{O_2}$ =

Answer: ____________________

e. Based on the above information, calculate the patient's pulmonary shunt.

$$\frac{\dot{Q}s}{\dot{Q}t} =$$

Answer: ____________________

14. What is the clinical significance of the following calculated shunts?

    a. Below 10%: ______________________________

    ____

    b. Between 10-20%: ______________________________

    ____

    ____

    c. Between 20 and 30%: ______________________________

    ____

    ____

    ____

    d. Greater than 30%: ______________________________

    ____

    ____

    ____

15. List three clinical factors that cause the calculation of pulmonary shunting to be unreliable.

    a. ______________________________

    b. ______________________________

    c. ______________________________

16. **Hypoxic Hypoxia** is defined as: ______________________________

    ____

    ____

17. List some conditions that can cause hypoxic hypoxia.

    a. ______________________________

    b. ______________________________

    c. ______________________________

18. **Anemic Hypoxia** is defined as: ____________________

19. List two conditions that cause anemic hypoxia.

a. ____________________

b. ____________________

20. **Circulatory hypoxia** is defined as: ____________________

21. List two major forms of circulatory hypoxia.

a. ____________________

b. ____________________

22. **Histotoxic hypoxia** is defined as: ____________________

23. Define **cyanosis**. ____________________

24. Define **polycythemia**. ____________________

CHAPTER EIGHT
CARBON DIOXIDE TRANSPORT
AND
ACID-BASE BALANCE

SECTION A

1. List the three ways that carbon dioxide is transported from the tissue cells to the lungs in the <u>plasma</u>.

    a. ______________________________

    b. ______________________________

    c. ______________________________

2. List the three ways that carbon dioxide is transported from the tissue cells to the lungs in the <u>red blood cells</u>.

    a. ______________________________

    b. ______________________________

    c. ______________________________

3. In what form is most of the carbon dioxide carried to the lungs?

    ANSWER: ____________________

4. The answer to the above question accounts for about _______ percent of the total amount of carbon dioxide transported to the lungs.

5. Using the following illustration, write the various chemical reaction(s) carbon dioxide goes through at the tissue sites to be transported to the lungs.

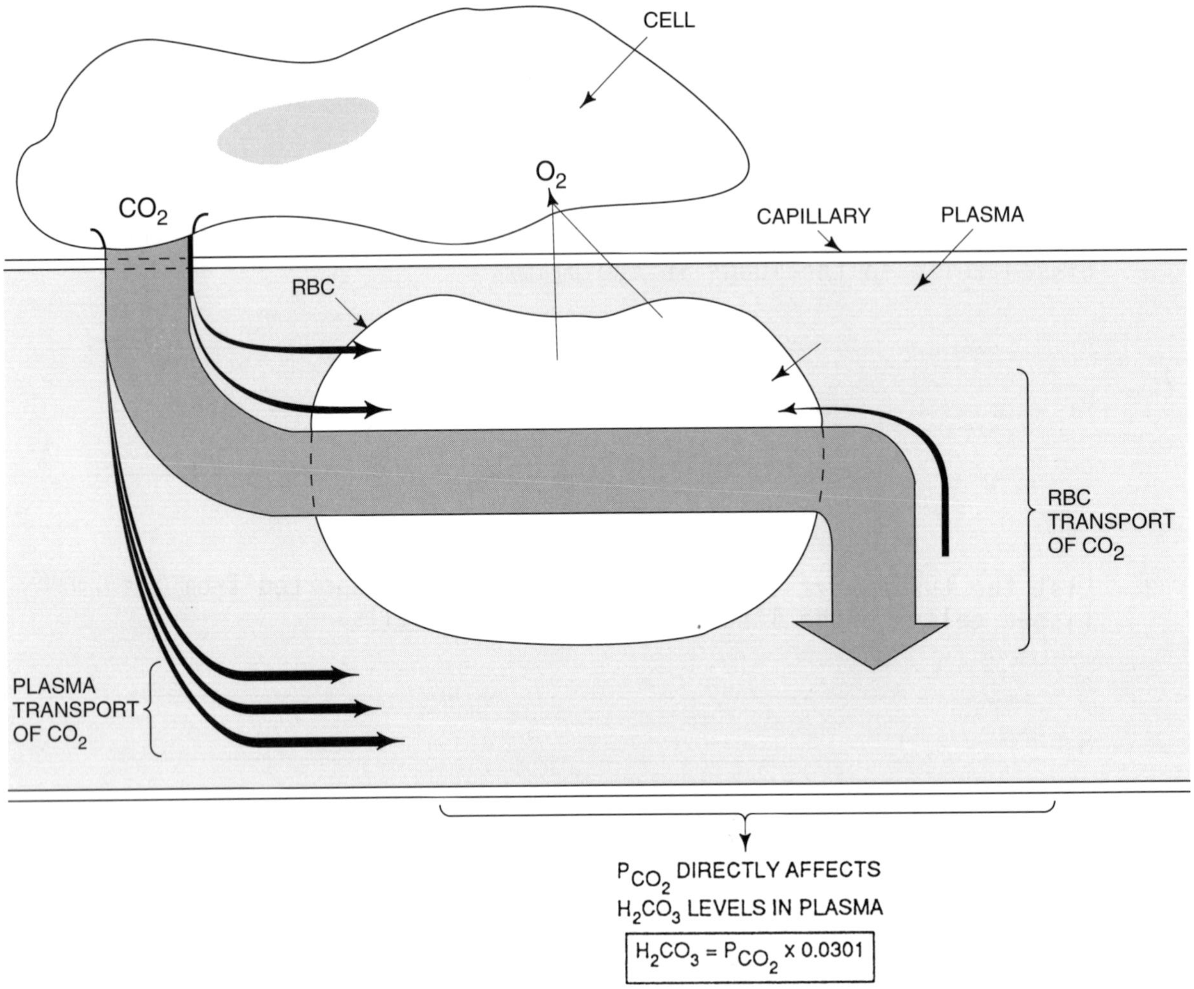

How CO_2 is converted to HCO_3^- at the tissue sites. Most of the CO_2 that is produced at the tissue cells is carried to the lungs in the form of HCO_3^-. CA = carbonic anhydrase.

6. Unlike the S-shaped oxygen dissociation curve, the carbon dioxide curve is much more ________________.

7. Using the following carbon dioxide dissociation curve nomogram, if the P_{CO_2} increases from 25 mm Hg to 40 mm Hg, the carbon

dioxide contents increases from ___________ Vol% to ________ Vol%.

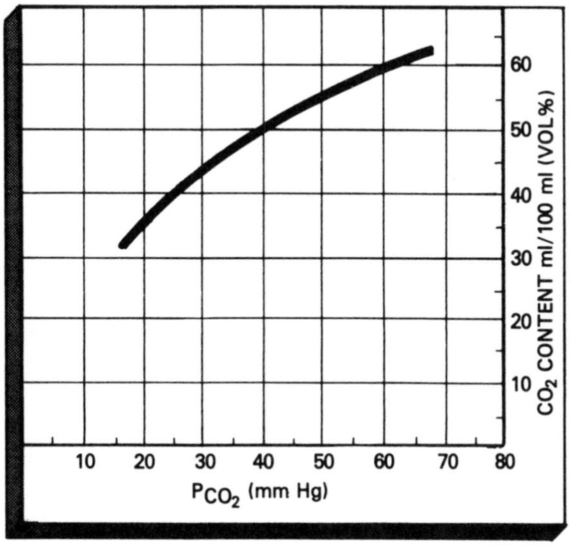

8. The fact that deoxygenated blood enhances the loading of carbon

dioxide is called the ____.

SECTION B

1. **Electrolytes** are: ____

____

____

2. A **buffer** is a: ____

____

____

____

3. A **strong acid** is an acid that: ______________________________

____

____

4. A **weak acid** is an acid that: ______________________________

____

____

5. A **strong base** is a base that: ______________________________

____

____

6. A **weak base** is a base that: ______________________________

____

____

7. A **dissociation constant** refers to: ______________________

____

____

____

8. In regard to the following equation, circle the portion of the equation that is in the dissociated state:

$$HA \rightleftharpoons [H^+] + [A^-]$$

9. A pH of 7 is ______________________.

10. A pH less than 7 is ____________________.

11. A pH greater than 7 is ____________________.

12. In chemistry, the pH is defined as: ______________________

____

____

13. The above definition of pH is written as:

pH =

14. A pH of 7 is equal to ______________ mole/L.

15. An <u>acid</u> is a substance that (______ accepts; ______ donates) $[H^+]$.

16. An <u>acid</u> is a substance that (______ increases; ______ decreases) the numerical value of the pH.

17. A <u>base</u> is a substance that (______ accepts; ______ donates) $[H^+]$.

18. A <u>base</u> is a substance that (______ increases; ______ decreases) the numerical value of the pH.

19. List the three mechanisms that maintain the narrow pH range.

a. ____

____

b. ____

____

c. ____

____

20. The most important buffer system in respiratory physiology is the

____ combination.

21. The **Henderson-Hasselbalch equation** uses the components of the $H_2CO_3^-/HCO_3^-$ system in the following way:

pH =

22. **pK** is derived from: ____

____

____

23. Normally, the pK is ____________________.

24. The normal HCO_3^- to $H_2CO_3^-$ ratio is __________ to __________.

25. An HCO_3^- to $H_2CO_3^-$ ratio of 17:1 means the pH is:

   a. normal
   b. less than normal
   c. greater than normal

26. An HCO_3^- to H_2CO_3 ratio of 26:1 means the pH is:

   a. normal
   b. less than normal
   c. greater than normal

SECTION C

1. During acute ventilatory failure (hypoventilation), the blood:

   a. P_{CO_2} (___ increase; ___ decrease; ___ remains the same)

   b. H_2CO_3 (___ increase; ___ decrease; ___ remains the same)

   c. HCO_3^- (___ increase; ___ decrease; ___ remains the same)

   d. HCO_3^- to H_2CO_3 ratio (___ increase; ___ decrease; ___ remains the same)

   e. pH (___ increase; ___ decrease; ___ remains the same)

2. In chronic ventilatory failure, the kidneys work to correct the pH status by:

   a. excreting HCO_3^-
   b. retaining H_2CO_3
   c. excreting H_2CO_3
   d. retaining HCO_3^-

3. In chronic ventilatory failure, partial or complete renal compensation can be verified when the HCO_3^- and pH readings on the $P_{CO_2}/HCO_3^-/pH$ nomogram are:

   a. greater than expected for a particular Pa_{CO_2}

   b. less than expected for a particular Pa_{CO_2}

4. During **acute alveolar hyperventilation** the blood:

   a. P_{CO_2} (___increases; ___ decreases; ___ remains the same)

   b. H_2CO_3 (___ increases; ___ decreases; ___ remains the same)

   c. HCO_3^- (___ increases; ___ decreases; ___ remains the same)

   d. HCO_3^- to H_2CO_3 ratio (___ increases; ___ decreases; ___ remains the same)

   e. pH (___ increases; ___ decreases; ___ remains the same)

5. In **chronic alveolar hyperventilation**, the kidneys work to correct the pH status by:

   a. excreting HCO_3^-
   b. retaining H_2CO_3
   c. excreting H_2CO_3
   d. retaining HCO_3^-

6. In chronic alveolar hyperventilation, partial or complete renal compensation can be verified when the HCO_3^- and pH readings are:

   a. greater than expected for a particular Pa_{CO_2}

   b. less than expected for a particular Pa_{CO_2}

7. True ___ False ___ As a general rule, the kidneys have a tendency to overcompensate for an abnormal pH.

8. When **metabolic acidosis** is present, the HCO_3^- and pH readings are:

   a. greater than expected for a particular Pa_{CO_2}

   b. less than expected for a particular Pa_{CO_2}

9. List three common causes of metabolic acidosis.

   a. ____

   b. ____

   c. ____

10. In response to a metabolic acidosis condition, the ventilatory rate:

    a. increases
    b. decreases
    c. remains the same

11. When **metabolic alkalosis** is present, the HCO_3^- and pH readings are:

    a. greater than expected for a particular Pa_{CO_2}

    b. less than expected for a particular Pa_{CO_2}

12. List five common causes of metabolic alkalosis.

    a. ____________________

    b. ____________________

    c. ____________________

    d. ____________________

    e. ____________________

13. Using the following $P_{CO_2}/HCO_3^-/pH$ nomogram, answer questions a through d:

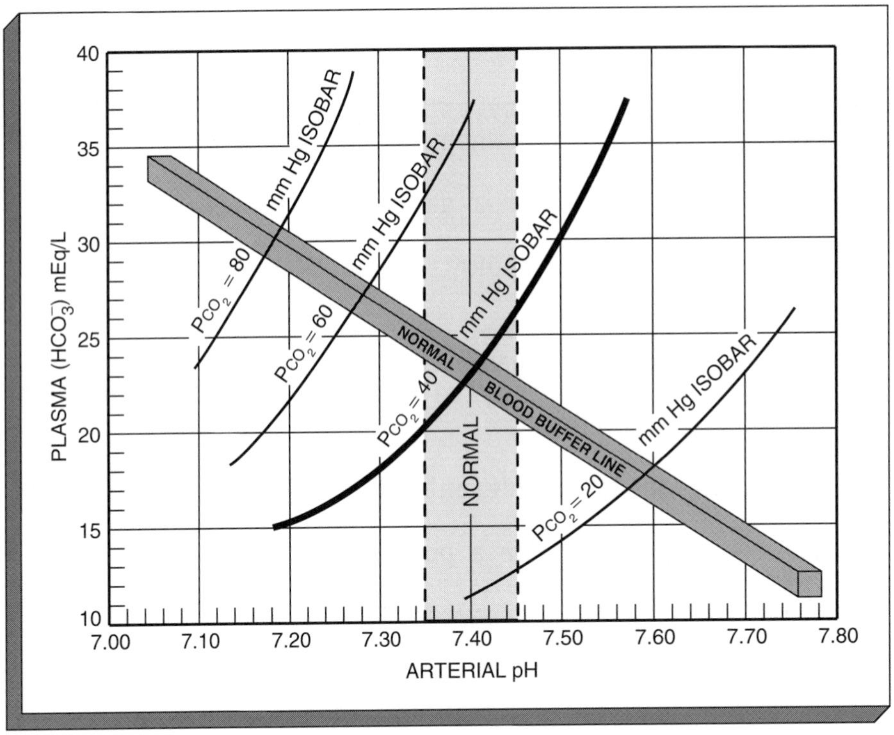

Nomogram of $Pc_{O_2}/HCO_3^-/pH$ relationship.

a. If a patient's ventilatory rate suddenly decreased, and the patient's Pa_{CO_2} increased to 70 mm Hg, what would be the expected pH and HCO_3^- changes?

ANSWER: pH ____________________

HCO_3^- ____________________

13. (continued)

b. If a patient's ventilatory rate suddenly increased, causing the patient's Pa_{CO_2} to decrease to 20 mm Hg, what would be the expected pH and HCO_3^- changes?

ANSWER: pH ________________

HCO_3^- ________________

c. Part I:

If a patient presents a pH of 7.2 and a Pa_{CO_2} of 60 mm Hg, does the patient have a metabolic or respiratory acid-base imbalance or a combination of both?

ANSWER: ____________________________

Part II:

Which does the above patient have; a base excess or a base deficit?

ANSWER: ____________________________

Part III:

In order to return the patient's pH back to 7.4, how much of a base excess or base deficit does the patient have?

ANSWER: ____________________________

d. Part I:

If a patient presents a pH of 7.52 and a Pa_{CO_2} of 25 mm Hg, does the patient have a metabolic or respiratory acid-base imbalance or a combination of both?

ANSWER: ____________________________

Part II:

Which does the patient have; a base excess or a base deficit?

ANSWER: ____________________________

Part III:

In order to return the patient's pH back to 7.4, how much of a base excess or base deficit does the patient have?

ANSWER: ____________________________

Chapter Nine
Ventilation - Perfusion Relationships

SECTION A

1. The normal alveolar ventilation is about _________ L/minute.

2. The normal pulmonary capillary blood flow is about _________ L/minute.

3. The average overall ventilation/perfusion ratio is

   _______ : _______ or _______.

4. In the normal individual in the upright position, the V/Q ratio in the upper lung region is (_________ higher; _________ lower) than 0.8.

5. In the normal individual in the upright position, the V/Q ratio in the lower lung region is (_________ higher; ________ lower) than 0.8.

6. In the upright lung, the V/Q ratio progressively (_________ increases; _________ decreases; _________ remains the same) from the top to the bottom.

7. The PA_{O_2} is determined by the balance between:

   a. ____

   ____

   b. ____

   ____

8. The PA_{CO_2} is determined by the balance between:

   a. ____

   ____

   ____

   b. ____

   ____

   ____

9. When the $\dot{V}/\dot{Q}$ ratio increases, the PA_{CO_2} decreases because: _____

____

____

____

10. When the $\dot{V}/\dot{Q}$ ratio increases, the PA_{O_2} increases because: _____

____

____

____

____

11. In the upright lung, an increased $\dot{V}/\dot{Q}$ ratio is found in the:

a. upper lung regions
b. middle lung regions
c. lower lung regions

12. When the $\dot{V}/\dot{Q}$ ratio decreases, the PA_{O_2} decreases because: _____

____

____

____

13. When the $\dot{V}/\dot{Q}$ ratio decreases, the PA_{CO_2} increases because: _____

____

____

____

14. In the upright lung, a decreased $\dot{V}/\dot{Q}$ ratio is found in the:

a. upper lung regions
b. middle lung regions
c. lower lung regions

15. In the upright lung, the Pc_{O_2} (_____ increases; _____ decreases; _____ remains the same) from the top to the bottom.

16. In the upright lung, the Pc_{CO_2} (_____ increases; _____ decreases; _____ remains the same) from the top to the bottom.

17. In the upright lung, the pH in the end-capillary blood (_____ increases; _____ decreases; _____ remains the same) from the top to the bottom.

18. **Internal respiration** is defined as: ______________________________

____

____

19. Normally, about ________ ml of oxygen are consumed by the tissue cells in one minute.

20. Normally, the tissue cells produce about ________ ml of carbon dioxide in one minute.

21. **Respiratory quotient** (RQ) is defined as the: ___________________

____

____

22. The respiratory quotient is expressed as:

RQ =

23. **External respiration** is defined as: ______________________________

____

____

24. **Respiratory exchange ratio** (RR) is defined as the: ____________

____

____

____

25. List some pulmonary disorders that increase the $\dot{V}/\dot{Q}$ ratio.

a. ____

____

b. ____

____

c. ____

____

d. ____

____

e. ____

____

26. List some pulmonary disorders that decrease the $\dot{V}/\dot{Q}$ ratio.

a. ____

____

b. ____

____

c. ____

____

CHAPTER TEN
CONTROL OF VENTILATION

SECTION A

1. It is now believed that the DRG and VRG neurons in the medulla oblongata are responsible for coordinating the intrinsic rhythmicity of respiration. DRG and VRG are abbreviations for the following:

   a. DRG:____

   b. VRG:____

2. The DRG consist chiefly of:

   a. Inspiratory neurons
   b. Expiratory neurons
   c. Inspiratory and Expiratory neurons

3. The VRG consist of:

   a. Inspiratory neurons
   b. Expiratory neurons
   c. Inspiratory and Expiratory neurons

4. Which of the following is activated only during heavy exercise or stress?

   a. DRG
   b. VRG

5. Where is the **apneustic center** located?

   ____

   ____

6. If unrestrained, the apneustic center causes:

   a. Prolonged expiration
   b. Prolonged inspiration

7. Which of the following suppress the function of the apneustic center?

   a. DRG
   b. Pneumotaxic center
   c. VRG

8. The respiratory components (DRG and VRG) of the medulla are primarily influenced by an excessive concentration of ________________.

9. Where are the **central chemoreceptors** located? ____________________

   ____

   ____

10. The **blood-brain barrier** is very permeable to __________ molecules, and relatively impermeable to ______ and ______ ions.

11. Write the chemical reaction that forms carbonic acid when CO_2 moves into the cerebrospinal fluid.

CO_2 +

12. How do the central chemoreceptors respond to the liberated [H+] produced in the above reaction?

____

____

____

____

13. In essence, the central chemoreceptors regulate ventilation through the (_____ direct; _____ indirect) effects of CO_2 on the: ______

____

14. The **peripheral chemoreceptors** are:______________________________

____

____

____

15. Where are the peripheral chemoreceptors located?_______________

____

____

____

16. When activated by a low Pa_{O_2}, the carotid bodies send neural impulses to the respiratory components of the medulla by way of the ______________________________ nerve; the aortic bodies send neural impulses to the medulla by way of the ________________ nerve.

17. Which of the following play a greater role in causing the ventilatory rate to increase in response to a decreased Pa_{O_2}?

a. Carotid bodies
b. Aortic bodies

18. At about what Pa_{O_2} level are the peripheral chemoreceptors significantly activated?

    Answer:________________

19. Suppression of the peripheral chemoreceptors is seen when the Pa_{O_2} falls below ______________________________.

20. Why are the peripheral chemoreceptors totally responsible for the control of ventilation when the Pa_{CO_2} level is chronically high?

    ____

    ____

    ____

    ____

    ____

    ____

    ____

21. In response to a chronically high CO_2 level, the sensitivity of the peripheral chemoreceptors:

    a. increases
    b. decreases
    c. remains the same

22. List some clinical conditions in which the P_{O_2} is normal, but the oxygen content is dangerously low.

    a. ____

    b. ____

    c. ____

23. List some other factors that stimulate the peripheral chemoreceptors.

    a. ____

    b. ____

    c. ____

    d. ____

    e. ____

24. In addition to an increase in ventilation, list some other responses that occur when the peripheral chemoreceptors are stimulated.

    a. ______________________________

    b. ______________________________

    c. ______________________________

    d. ______________________________

    e. ______________________________

SECTION B

1. What activates the **Hering-Breuer reflex?**______________________________

   ____

2. When activated, the Hering-Breuer reflex cause(s):______________________________

   ____

3. What activates the **deflation reflex?**______________________________

   ____

4. When activated, the deflation reflex cause(s):______________________________

   ____

5. What activates the **irritant reflex?**______________________________

   ____

   ____

6. Where are the irritant receptors located?______________________________

   ____

7. When activated, the irritant reflex cause(s):______________________________

   ____

8. Where are the **J receptors** located?______________________________

____

9. What activates the J receptors?

   a. ____

   b. ____

   c. ____

   d. ____

   e. ____

   f. ____

10. When activated, the J receptors cause(s):______________________

____

11. In response to an elevated systemic blood pressure, the **aortic and carotid sinus baroreceptors** cause:

____

____

12. In response to a reduced systemic blood pressure, the aortic and carotid sinus baroreceptors cause:

____

____

13. How does the following affect ventilation?

   a. A sudden cold stimulus.______________________________________

   ____

   ____

   b. A sudden pain.____

   ____

   ____

c. Irritation of the pharynx or larynx.________________________

____

____

____

d. Stretching of the anal sphincter.___________________________

____

____

e. Light pressure applied to the thorax.________________________

____

____

Chapter Eleven
Cardiopulmonary Physiology
of
The Fetus and the Newborn

SECTION A

1. List the four periods of lung development during fetal life.

   a. ______________________________

   b. ______________________________

   c. ______________________________

   d. ______________________________

2. The lungs first appear as a small bud arising from the esophagus on the ______ day of embryonic life.

3. By the 16th week of gestation, there are about ______ generations of bronchial airways.

4. By the _____ week of gestation, the air-blood interface between the alveoli and the pulmonary capillaries and the quantity of pulmonary surfactant are usually sufficient to support life.

5. Anatomically, the placenta consists of about 15 to 20 segments called

   __________________________.

6. Label and color the following anatomic structures of the placenta:

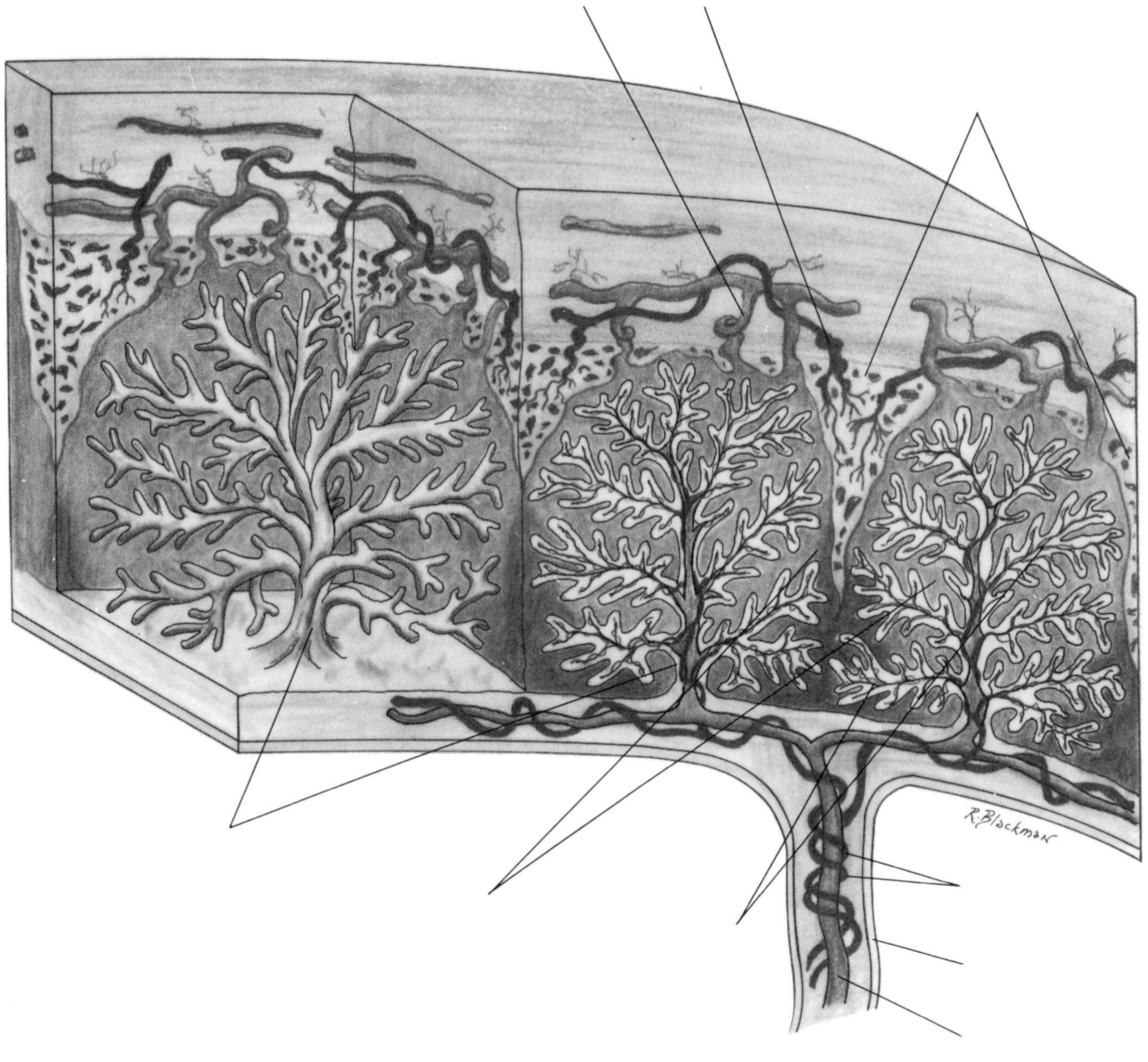

Anatomic structure of the cotyledon of the placenta.

7. Deoxygenated blood is carried from the fetus to the placenta by way of two ____.

8. Normally, the P_{O_2} in the umbilical arteries is about ______ mm Hg and the P_{CO_2} is about ________ mm Hg.

9. Explain why the maternal blood P_{CO_2} is frequently lower than expected during the last trimester of pregnancy.

____

____

____

____

10. Once in the intervillous space, oxygen transfers from the maternal to fetal blood because of the:

a. ____

____

b. ____

____

c. ____

____

11. As oxygenated fetal blood flows out of the chorionic villi, the P_{O_2} is about _______ mm Hg, and the P_{CO_2} is about _______ mm Hg.

12. Oxygenated fetal blood flows out of the chorionic villi and returns to the fetus by way of the ______________________________.

13. List the three factors thought to be responsible for the wide variance between the maternal and fetal P_{O_2} and P_{CO_2}.

a. ____

____

b. ____

____

c. ____

____

SECTION B

1. As oxygenated blood from the placenta returns to the fetus, about one-half of the blood enters the liver of the fetus and the rest enters the inferior vena cava by flowing through the ___________ _______________________________.

2. Once in the right atrium of the fetus, most of the blood flows directly into the left atrium through the ______________________.

3. The blood in the left atrium of the fetus enters the ____________ _____________________________ and is then pumped primarily to the __________________ and ___________________.

4. Most of the fetal blood that passes into the pulmonary artery from the right ventricle bypasses the lungs by passing through the __________________________ and flows directly into the _________________.

5. Approximately ______ percent of the fetal circulation passes through the lungs and returns to the left atrium via the _________________ _______________________.

6. The Pa_{O_2} in the descending aorta is about ________ mm Hg.

MATCHING:

7. Directions: In Column A, match the order (i.e., from first to last) in which fetal blood passes through the structures in Column B.

Column A	Column B
Order	Structure
1. ________	A. Common Iliac Arteries
2. ________	B. External and Internal Iliacs
3. _______	C. Ductus Arteriosus
4. _______	D. Umbilical Arteries
5. _______	E. Ductus Vensous

8. Describe the changes the special structures of the fetal circulation go through after birth.

   a. ______________________________

   ____

   ____

   b. ______________________________

   ____

   ____

   c. ______________________________

   ____

   ____

   d. ______________________________

   ____

   ____

   e. ______________________________

   ____

   ____

   f ______________________________

   ____

   ____

SECTION C

1. Describe the three primary mechanisms that remove the fluid from the fetal lungs during the first 24 hours of life.

   a. ______________________________

   ____

   ____

   b. ______________________________

   ____

   ____

c. ____

____

____

2. About ________ million primitive alveoli are present at birth.

3. The number of alveoli continue to increase until about __________ years of age.

4. List some of the stimuli that cause the infant to take its first breath at birth.

   a. ______________________________

   b. ______________________________

   c. ______________________________

5. During the first breath, it is estimated that the infant's intrapleural pressure decreases to about _______ cm H_2O before any air enters the lungs.

6. About ______ ml of air enters the lungs during the first breath.

7. The average lung compliance (C_L) of the newborn is about

   ______________________________.

8. The average airway resistance (R_{aw}) of the newborn is about

   ______________________________.

9. List the two major mechanisms that account for the decreased pulmonary vascular resistance when an infant inhales for the first time.

   a. ____

   ____

   ____

   b. ____

   ____

   ____

10. Describe the mechanism that causes the foramen ovale to close functionally at birth.

____

____

____

____

____

____

____

11. At birth, the newborn's P_{O_2} must increase to more than ________ to ________ mm Hg in order for the ductus arteriosus to close.

12. Describe the meaning of persistent pulmonary hypertension of the neonate (PPHN).

____

____

____

____

13. Persistent pulmonary hypertension of the neonate was previously known as ____.

14. List other substances that are released at birth that are believed to contribute to the constriction of the ductus arteriosus.

a. ____

b. ____

c. ____

15. Although inhibited during fetal life, the ________________ and ________________ chemoreceptors play a major role in activating the first breath at birth.

16. Stimulation of the newborn's trigeminal nerve causes the infant's respiration and heart rate to ________________.

17. Stimulation of the pre-term infant's irritant reflex is commonly followed by ______________________________.

18. Stimulation of the term infant's irritant reflex causes ______________ ______________________________.

19. The Head Paradoxical Reflex is: ______________________________
____
____

20. Compare and contrast the approximate lung volumes and capacities of the newborn.

TABLE 11–1. Approximate Lung Volumes and Capacities of the Newborn

Tidal volume (V_T)	Vital capacity (VC)
Residual volume (RV)	Functional residual capacity (FRC)
Expiratory reserve volume (ERV)	Inspiratory capacity (IC)
Inspiratory reserve volume (IRV)	Total lung capacity (TLC)

21. Write the normal vital sign ranges of the newborn.

TABLE 11–2. Normal Vital Sign Ranges of the Newborn

Respiratory rate (RR)
Heart rate (HR)
Blood pressure (BP)

Chapter Twelve
Renal Failure
And Its Influence On
The Cardiopulmonary System

SECTION A

1. Label and color the following structures that form the **kidney**.

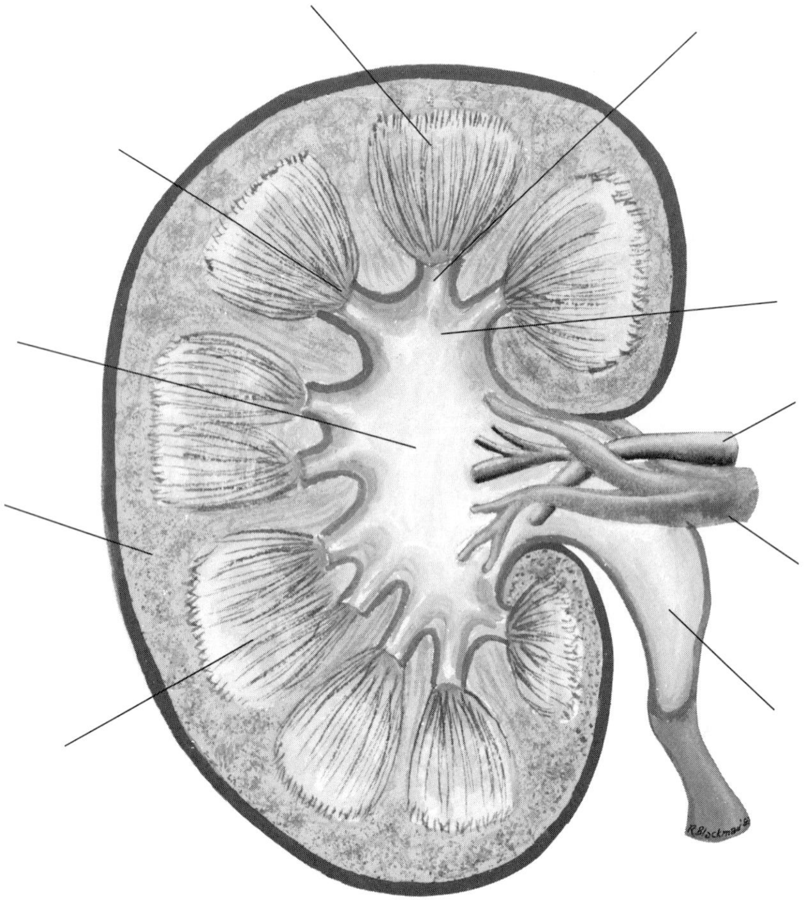

2. Label and color the following structures of the **nephron**.

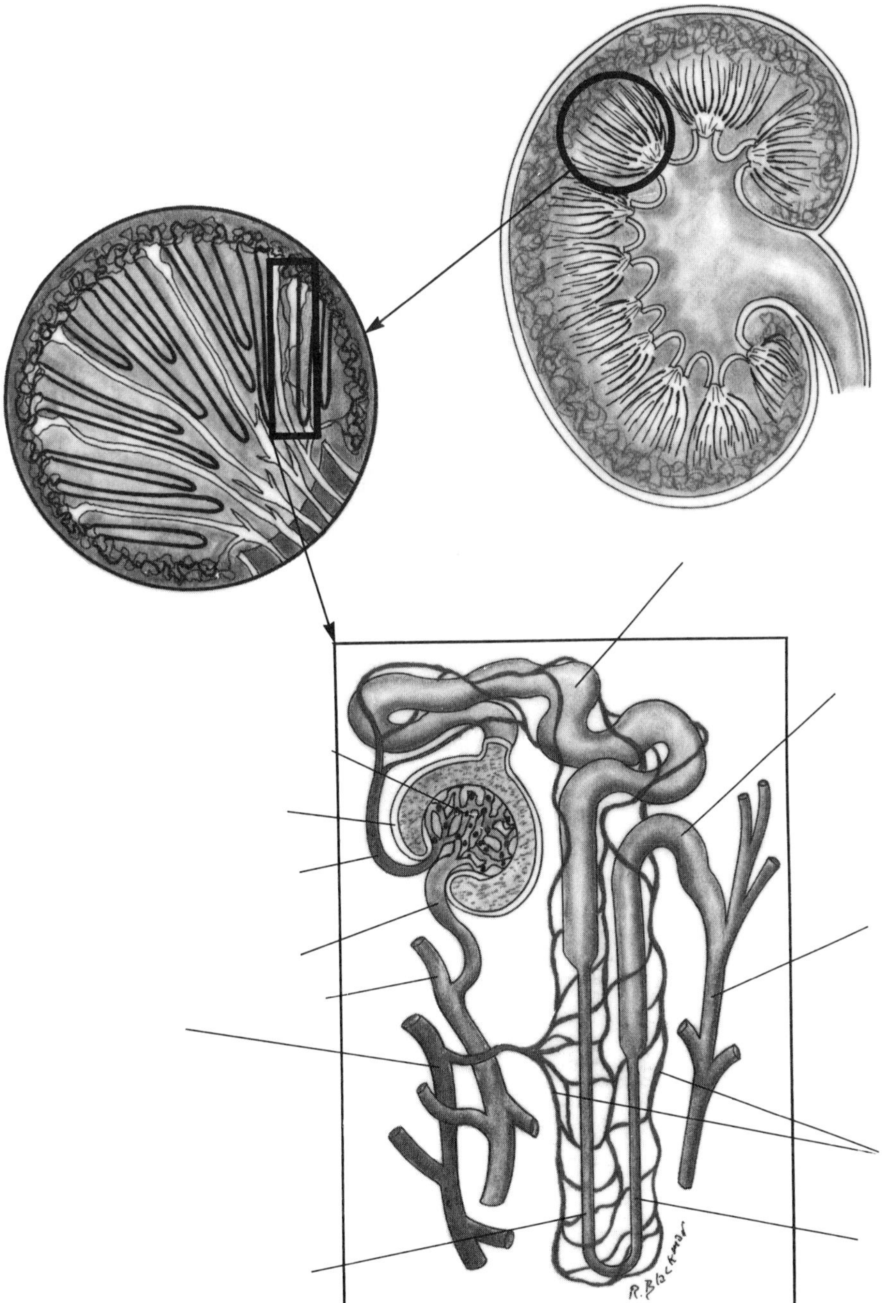

The nephron.

3. Label and color the following **blood vessels** of the kidney.

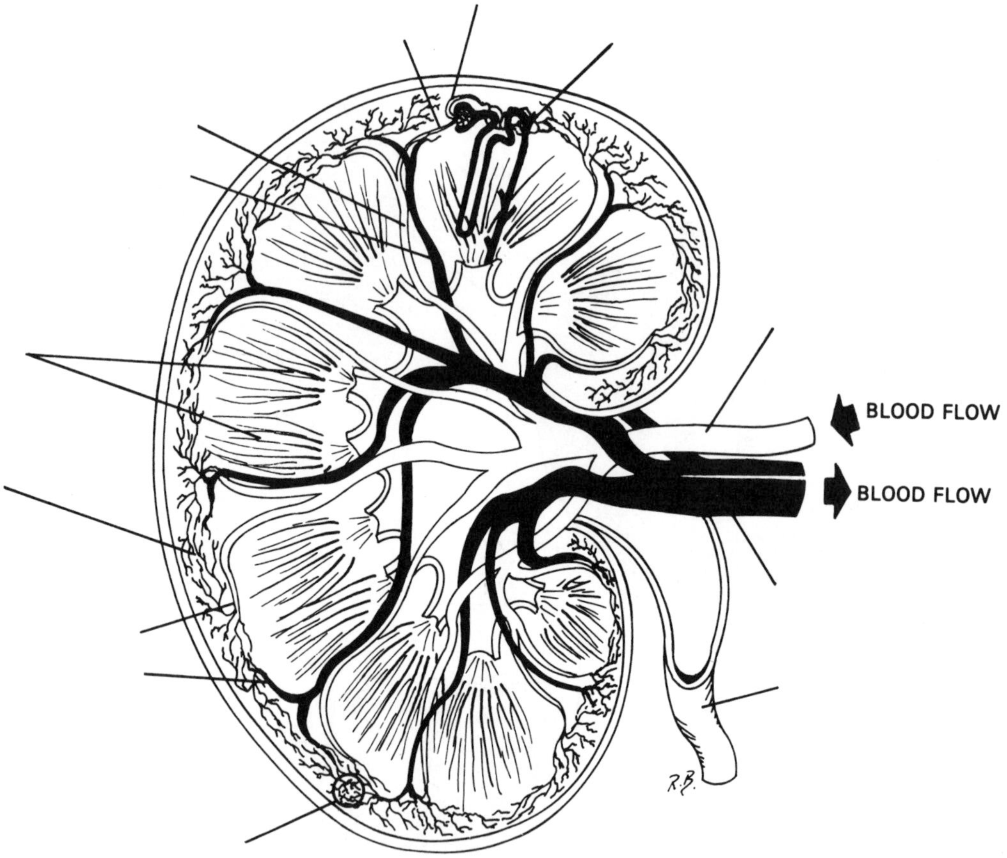

Blood vessels of the kidney.

SECTION B

1. Compare and contrast the forces of glomerular filtration.

TABLE 12–1. Forces of Glomerular Filtration

FACTORS	FORCE
Enhances Filtration	
Glomerular capillary blood pressure	
Opposes Filtration	
Fluid pressure in Bowman's capsule	
Osmotic force (caused by the protein concentration difference)	________
Net Filtration Pressure	

2. List the four major structures responsible for tubular reabsorption.

   a. ____________________

   b. ____________________

   c. ____________________

3. The bulk of **tubular reabsorption** occurs in the ____________________

   ____________________.

4. **Tubular secretion** is the mechanism by which ____________________

   ____

   ____

   ____

   ____

5. The most important substances transported into the tubules by means of secretion are ________________ and ______________ ions.

6. The kidneys control the concentration and volume of urine by virtue of the following two mechanisms:

   a. ____

   b. ____

   ____

7. The **juxtamedullary nephrons** are located deep into the __________ ________________________.

8. The normal osmolality of the glomerular filtrate is approximately _________ mOsm/L.

9. The osmolality of the interstitial fluid ranges from about _______ mOsm/L in the cortex to about _______ mOsm/L as the juxtamedullary nephron descends into the renal medulla.

10. ADH is produced in the ____________________ and released by the _________________________.

11. When the atrial blood volume and pressure increase, the production of ADH:

    a. increases
    b. decreases
    c. remains the same

12. When the atrial blood volume and pressure decrease, the production of ADH:

    a. increases
    b. decreases
    c. remains the same

13. When the production of ADH decreases, the volume of urine (_____ increases; _____ decreases).

14. When the production of ADH increases, the volume of urine (_____ increases; _____ decreases).

15. The urine produced by the healthy kidney has a specific gravity of about _________ to _________.

16. List some of the more important ions regulated by the kidneys.

    a. ______________________________

    b. ______________________________

    c. ______________________________

17. When the extracellular fluid becomes too acidic, the kidneys excrete ______________ ions into the urine.

18. When the extracellular fluid becomes too alkaline, the kidneys excrete (primarily) ______________________________ into the urine.

19. The two major mechanisms responsible for maintaining an individual's blood volume at a consistent level are:

    a. ______________________________

    b. ______________________________

SECTION C

1. List some congenital renal disorders.

    a. ______________________________

    b. ______________________________

    c. ______________________________

2. Urinary tract infections are seen more often in (____ men; ____ women).

3. List some factors that predispose an individual to urinary flow obstruction.

    a. ______________________________

    b. ______________________________

    c. ______________________________

    d. ______________________________

    e. ______________________________

4. List some causes of kidney inflammation.

   a. ______________________________

   b. ______________________________

   c. ______________________________

5. Name the form of cancer that accounts for about 70% of all cancers of early childhood.

   Answer ______________________.

6. List some common prerenal causes of renal failure.

   a. ______________________________

   b. ______________________________

   c. ______________________________

   d. ______________________________

7. What is one of the early clinical manifestations of **prerenal failure**?

   Answer ______________________________.

8. List the five categories of **renal** abnormalities that cause renal failure.

   a. ______________________________

   b. ______________________________

   c. ______________________________

   d. ______________________________

   e. ______________________________

9. List some **postrenal** abnormalities that cause renal failure.

   a. ______________________________

   b. ______________________________

10. Positive pressure ventilation (_____ increases; _____ decreases) urinary output.

11. Negative pressure ventilation (_____ increases; _____ decreases) urinary output.

12. When positive pressure ventilation causes the blood volume and, therefore, the pressure in the atria to decrease, the release of ADH:

    a. increases
    b. decreases
    c. remains the same

13. When the concentration of ADH increases, the amount of urine formed:

    a. increases
    b. decreases
    c. remains the same

14. Hypertension and edema develop in renal failure because of the

    kidney's inability to excrete ______________________.

15. When the kidneys fail, metabolic acidosis develops because the following:

    a. H^+ (_____ increases; _____ decreases)

    b. K^+ (_____ increases; _____ decreases)

    c. HCO_3^- (_____ increases; _____ decreases)

16. **Hypochloremia** causes:

    a. acidosis
    b. alkalosis

17. **Hypokalemia** causes:

    a. acidosis
    b. alkalosis

18. **Hyperchloremia** causes:

    a. acidosis
    b. alkalosis

19. **Hyperkalemia** causes:

    a acidosis
    b. alkalosis

20. What two mechanisms contribute to the anemia seen in chronic renal failure?

    a. ____

    ____

    ____

    ____

b. ______________________________

21. Why do patients with chronic renal failure have a tendency to bleed?

____

22. Why is pericarditis seen in about 50% of persons with chronic renal failure?

____

CHAPTER THIRTEEN
AGING
AND ITS INFLUENCE ON
THE CARDIOPULMONARY SYSTEM

SECTION A

1. The growth and development of the lungs is essentially complete by about __________ years of age.

2. Most of the pulmonary function indices reach their maximum level between __________ and __________ years of age.

3. With aging, the elastic recoil of the lungs (_____ increases; _____ decreases; _____ remains the same), and the lung compliance (_____ increases; _____ decreases; _____ remains the same).

4. With aging, identify what changes occur with the following lung volumes and capacities:

   a. RV (_____ increases; _____ decreases; _____ remains the same)

   b. IC (_____ increases; _____ decreases; _____ remains the same)

   c. VC (_____ increases; _____ decreases; _____ remains the same)

   d. TLC (_____ increases; _____ decreases; _____ remains the same)

   e. RV/TLC (_____ increases; _____ decreases; _____ remains the same)

   f. FRC (_____ increases; _____ decreases; _____ remains the same)

   g. ERV (_____ increases; _____ decreases; _____ remains the same)

5. With aging, identify what changes occur with the following **dynamic maneuvers** of ventilation.

   a. FVC (_____ increases; _____ decreases; _____ remains the same)

   b. PEFR (_____ increases; _____ decreases; _____ remains the same)

   c. $FEF_{25\%-75\%}$ (_____ increases; _____ decreases; _____ remains the same)

   d. FEV_1 (_____ increases; _____ decreases; _____ remains the same)

   e. FEV_1/FVC Ratio (_____ increases; _____ decreases; _____ remains the same)

   f. MVV (_____ increases; _____ decreases; _____ remains the same)

6. With aging, identify what changes occur with the following components of the respiratory system.

   a. Pulmonary Diffusing Capacity (_____ increases; _____ decreases; _____ remains the same)

   b. Alveolar Deadspace Ventilation (_____ increases; _____ decreases; _____ remains the same)

   c. $P(A-a)_{O_2}$ (_____ increases; _____ decreases; _____ remains the same)

   d. Pa_{O_2} (_____ increases; _____ decreases; _____ remains the same)

   e. Pa_{CO_2} (_____ increases; _____ decreases; _____ remains the same)

   f. HCO_3^- (_____ increases; _____ decreases; _____ remains the same)

   g. pH (_____ increases; _____ decreases; _____ remains the same)

   h. $C(a-\bar{v})_{O_2}$ (_____ increases; _____ decreases; _____ remains the same)

   i. Hemoglobin Concentration (_____ increases; _____ decreases; _____ remains the same)

7. With aging, the ventilatory response to both hypoxia and hypercapnia:

   a. increases
   b. decreases
   c. remains the same

8. With aging, the maximal oxygen uptake ($\dot{V}_{O_2\ max}$):

   a. increases
   b. decreases
   c. remains the same

9. With aging, the elasticity of the heart:

   a. increases
   b. decreases
   c. remains the same

10. With aging, the work of the heart:

    a. increases
    b. decreases
    c. remains the same

11. With aging, the heart rate increase in response to stress:

    a. increases
    b. decreases
    c. remains the same

12. What is the maximum heart rate for a 70-year-old?

Answer ______________________.

13. With aging, identify what changes develop with the following components of the cardiovascular system.

a. Stroke volume (___ increases; ____ decreases; ____ remains the same)

b. Cardiac output (____ increases; ____ decreases; ____ remains the same)

c. Resting pulse pressure (_____ increases; _____ decreases; _____ remains the same)

d. Systolic blood pressure (_____ increases; _____ decreases; _____ remains the same)

e. Peripheral vascular resistance (_____ increases; _____ decreases; _____ remains the same)

Chapter Fourteen
Exercise
And Its Effects On
The Cardiopulmonary System

SECTION A

1. During heavy exercise:

   a. Alveolar ventilation may increase as much as ________-fold.

   b. Oxygen diffusion capacity may increase as much as _______-fold.

   c. Cardiac output may increase as much as _______-fold.

   d. Muscle blood flow may increase as much as _______-fold.

   e. Oxygen consumption may increase as much as _______-fold.

   f. Heat production may increase as much as _______-fold.

2. Muscle training can increase muscle size and strength _______ to ________ percent.

3. The efficiency of intracellular metabolism may increase by __________ to __________ percent.

4. The size of the heart chambers and the heart mass of well-trained athletes may be increased by ___________ percent.

5. The point at which anaerobic metabolism develops is called ______________ ___________________.

6. It has been suggested that the increased ventilation seen in exercise is caused by the following:

   a. ____
   ____
   ____

   b. ____
   ____
   ____

   c. ____
   ____
   ____

SECTION B

1. During strenuous exercise, an adult alveolar ventilation can increase to:

   a. 40 liters per minute
   b. 60 liters per minute
   c. 80 liters per minute
   d. 100 liters per minute
   e. 120 liters per minute

2. During exercise, the increased alveolar ventilation is caused mainly by an increased __________ of ventilation, rather than an increased _________ of ventilation.

3. During very heavy exercise, both an increased ________ and ________ of ventilation is seen.

4. During very heavy exercise, the tidal volume is usually about what percent of the vital capacity?

   a. 10%
   b. 20%
   c. 30%
   d. 40%
   e. 50%

5. There are three distinct consecutive breathing patterns seen during mild and moderate exercise.

   a. The first stage is characterized by ______________________________

      ____

      ____

      ____

   b. The second stage is typified by ______________________________

      ____

      ____

      ____

   c. During the third stage, ______________________________________

      ____

      ____

      ____

6. The maximum alveolar ventilation generated during heavy exercise under normal conditions is about ____ to ____ percent of the maximum voluntary ventilation.

7. At rest, normal oxygen consumption ($\dot{V}_{02}$) is about _____ ml per minute.

8. During exercise, the skeletal muscles may account for more than ________ percent of the ($\dot{V}_{02}$).

9. The PaO_2 remains constant during:

   I. Mild exercise
   II. Moderate exercise
   III. Heavy exercise

   a. I only
   b. I and II only
   c. I, II, and III

10. It has been shown that the increased oxygen diffusion capacity results from the ______________________________________ during exercise.

11. During exercise, the $P(A-a)_{O_2}$ remains essentially constant until what percent of the maximal oxygen consumption is reached?

    a. 10%
    b. 20%
    c. 30%
    d. 40%
    e. 50%

SECTION C

1. These essential physiologic responses must occur in order for the circulatory system to supply the working muscles with an adequate amount of blood. These are:

   a. ______________________________

   b. ______________________________

   c. ______________________________

2. The two circulatory effects of the sympathetic discharge are:

   a. ______________________________

   ____

   ____

   ____

   b. ______________________________

   ____

   ____

   ____

3. The increased oxygen demands during exercise are met almost entirely by

   ______________________________.

4. The increased cardiac output during exercise results from:

   a. ______________________________

   b. ______________________________

   c. ______________________________

5. The increased stroke volume during exercise is primarily due to ________

   __________________ in the working muscles.

6. The ability of the heart to accommodate the increased venous return and, subsequently, increased cardiac output is due to the ______________ mechanism.

7. The maximum heart rate for a 55-year-old is about ______________.

8. When the stroke volume decreases, the heart rate (________ increases; ________ decreases; ________ remains the same), and when the stroke volume increases, the heart rate (________ increases; ________ decreases; ________ remains the same).

9. The stroke volume is influenced by:

   a. ______________________________

   ____

   b. ______________________________

   ____

   c. ______________________________

   ____

10. The body's ability to increase the heart rate and stroke volume during exercise progressively (_______ increases; _______ decreases) with age.

11. There is almost always an increase in arterial blood pressure during exercise because:

   a. ______________________________

   ____

   ____

   b. ______________________________

   ____

   ____

   c. ______________________________

   ____

   ____

12. As oxygen consumption and cardiac output increase during exercise, the pulmonary:

   a. Systolic pressure (___ increases; ___ decreases; ___ remains the same)

   b. Diastolic pressure (___ increases; ___ decreases; ___ remains the same)

   c. Arterial (mean) pressure (___ increases; ___ decreases; ___ remains the same)

   d. Wedge pressure (___ increases; ___ decreases; ___ remains the same)

13. The dilation of the blood vessels in the working muscles is caused primarily by ______________________________ acting on the arterioles.

14. During very heavy exercise the increased ________________________ accounts for a much greater proportion of the increased cardiac output than the ______________________________.

15. The stroke volume reaches its maximum when the maximum cardiac output is only at approximately _______ percent.

16. After the stroke volume reaches its maximum, any further increase in cardiac output is soley due to an ______________________________.

17. Maximum exercise taxes the respiratory system only about ____ percent of maximum.

18. List the symptoms that, collectively, are referred to as heat stroke.

____

____

____

____

____

____

19. The primary treatment of heat stroke consists of the following:

a. ______________________________

____

b. ______________________________

____

c. ______________________________

____

d. ______________________________

____

20. List the four phase(s) of the cardiovascular rehabilitation process:

a. Phase I:______________________________

____

b. Phase II:______________________________

____

c. Phase III:______________________________

____

d. Phase IV:______________________________

____

Chapter Fifteen High Altitude And Its Effects On The Cardiopulmonary System

SECTION A

1. The barometric pressure is about half the sea level value of 760 mm Hg at an altitude of ___________ feet.

2. One of the most prominent features of acclimatization is _____________

   ____.

3. In lowlanders who ascend to high altitudes, the RBC's increased for about _____________ before the production rate levels off.

4. People who live at high altitudes commonly demonstrate:

   a. Mild respiratory acidosis

   b. Normal arterial blood gas values

   c. Mild respiratory alkalosis

5. The oxygen diffusion capacity of lowlanders who are acclimatized to high altitude:

   a. increases
   b. decreases
   c. remains the same

6. The oxygen diffusion capacity of high-altitudes natives is about _______ ____________________ than predicted.

7. At high altitude, the alveolar arterial PO_2 difference $[P(A-a)O_2]$:

   a. increases
   b. decreases
   c. remains the same

8. At high altitude, the overall ventilation-perfusion ratio improves in response to the (____ increased; ____ decreased) pulmonary arterial blood pressure.

9. In individuals, who have acclimatized to high altitude, and in high-altitude natives, cardiac output:

   a. increases
   b. decreases
   c. remains the same

10. As an individual ascends, the pulmonary vascular system:

    a. constricts
    b. dilates
    c. remains the same

11. In high-altitude natives, the concentration of myoglobin in skeletal muscles:

    a. increases
    b. decreases
    c. remains the same

SECTION B

1. Acute mountain sickness is characterized by: ____________________________

   ____

   ____

   ____

2. The symptoms of acute mountain sickness are generally most severe on the:

   ____

   ____

3. Although the exact cause of high-altitude pulmonary edema is not fully understood, it may be associated with pulmonary (____ vasoconstriction; ____ vasodilation), and with a/an (____ increased; ____ decreased) permeability of the pulmonary capillaries.

4. High-altitude cerebral edema is characterized by: ______________________

   ____

   ____

   ____

5. Chronic mountain sickness is characterized by: _________________________

   ____

   ____

   ____

Chapter Sixteen High-Pressure Environments And Their Effect On The Cardiopulmonary System

---

SECTION A

1. For every 33 feet below the water surface, the pressure increases ______ ______________________ .

2. PART I

   If an individual fully inhales to a total lung capacity of 5.5 liters at sea level, and dives to a depth of 99 feet, the lungs will be compressed to about:

   Answer ______________________________

   PART II

   What is the pressure within the above diver's lungs?

   Answer ______________________________

3. The maximum time of a breath-hold dive is a function of:

   a. ______________________________

   ____

   b. ______________________________

   ____

4. In regard to the PCO_2, the so-called respiratory drive "breaking point" is about ____________ mm Hg.

5. The so-called CO_2 paradox occurs as a diver (____ descends; ____ ascends;) and the O_2 paradox occurs as the diver (____ descends; ____ ascends).

6. The fall in PAO_2 as a diver returns to the surface is known as the ______

   ______________________.

7. The dive response consists of:

   a. ______________________________

   b. ______________________________

   c. ______________________________

8. List some of the signs and symptoms collectively referred to a decompression sickness.

   a. ______________________________

   b. ______________________________

   c. ______________________________

   d. ______________________________

   e. ______________________________

9. Identify indications for hyperbaric oxygenation for the following clinical conditions.

TABLE 16–1. Indications for Hyperbaric Oxygenation
GAS DISEASES
VASCULAR INSUFFICIENCY STATES
INFECTIONS
DEFECTS IN OXYGEN TRANSPORT

10. Hyperbaric oxygen is effective in the treatment of carbon monoxide poisoning. The administration of hyperbaric oxygen:

    a. ____

    ____

    ____

    ____

    b. ____

    ____

    ____

    ____

    c. ____

    ____

    ____

    ____

11. Breathing 100% oxygen at one atmosphere changes the HbCO half-life, to less than ____________________.

ANSWERS

THE QUESTION NUMBERS REFER TO THE QUESTIONS IN THIS WORKBOOK. THE REFERENCE NUMBER REFERS TO THE TEXTBOOK CARDIOPULMONARY ANATOMY AND PHYSIOLOGY: ESSENTIALS FOR RESPIRATORY CARE, 2ND ED.

Chapter One
THE ANATOMY OF THE RESPIRATORY SYSTEM
Answers

SECTION A

1. (ref. pg. 8)
2. a. to act as a conductor of air
   b. to prevent foreign materials from entering the tracheobronchial tree
   c. serve as an important area involved in speech and smell (ref. pg. 7)
3. a. filter
   b. humidity (ref. pg. 7)
   c. warm
4. (ref. pg. 9)
5. (ref. pg. 10)
6. pseudostratified ciliated columnar (ref. pg. 8)
7. a. superior nasal turbinates
   b. middle nasal turbinates
   c. inferior nasal turbinates (ref. pg. 9)
8. (ref. pg. 12)
9. levator veli platinum (ref. pg. 10)
10. stratified squamous (ref. pg. 10)
11. palatoglossal, palatopharyngeal (ref. pg. 10)
12. pseudostratified ciliated columnar (ref. pg. 12)
13. eustachian tube (ref. pg. 12)
14. stratified squamous (ref. pg. 13)
15. stratified squamous (ref. pg. 13)
16. (ref. pg. 13)

SECTION B

1. a. acts as a passageway of air between the pharynx and the trachea
   b. works as a protective mechanism against the aspiration of solid and liquids
   c. generates sounds for speech (ref. pg. 15)
2. (ref. pg. 14)
3. (ref. pg. 16)
4. vocal ligament (ref. pg. 16)
5. thyroid cartilage (ref. pg. 16)
6. rima glottidis or glottis (ref. pg. 16)
7. stratified squamous (ref. pg. 16)
8. pseudostratified ciliated columnar (ref. pg. 16)
9. Valsalva's maneuver (ref. pg. 19)

10. (ref. pg. 18)
11. (ref. pg. 17)

Section C

1. a. epithelial lining
   b. lamina propria
   c. cartilaginous layer (ref. pg. 19)
2. pseudostratified ciliated columnar (ref. pg. 19)
3. submucosal glands (ref. pg. 20)
4. sol layer, gel layer (ref. pg. 20)
5. (ref. pg. 23)
6. a. cigarette smoke
   b. dehydration
   c. positive pressure ventilation
   d. endotracheal suctioning
   e. high inspired oxygen concentration
   f. hypoxia
   g. atmospheric pollutants
   h. general anesthetics
   i. parasympatholytics (ref. pgs. 21, 22)
7. a. histamine
   b. heparin
   c. slow-reacting substance of anaphylaxis
   d. platelet-activating factor
   e. eosinophilic chemotactic factors of anaphylaxis (ref. pgs. 24, 25)
8. 11 to 13, 1.5 to 2.5 (ref. pg. 26)
9. carina (ref. pg. 27)
10. 25, 40 to 60 (ref. pg. 27)
11. terminal bronchioles (ref. pg. 28)
12. increases (ref. pgs. 29, 30)
13. terminal bronchioles (ref. pg. 30)
14. mediastinal lymph nodes, the pulmonary nerves, muscular pulmonary arteries and veins, a portion of the esophagus, some visceral pleura (ref. pg. 31)
15. azygos, hemiazygos, intercostal veins (ref. pg. 31)
16. bronchopulmonary anastomoses (ref. pg. 31)

SECTION D

1. a. respiratory
   b. alveolar
   c. alveolar (ref. pg. 31)
2. (ref. pg. 32)
3. (ref. pg. 33)
4. 300 (ref. pg. 31)
5. 70 (ref. pg. 31)
6. respiratory bronchioles, alveolar ducts, and alveolar clusters (ref. pg. 31)
7. 130,000 (ref. pg. 31)

8. a. acinus
   b. terminal respiratory unit
   c. lung parenchyma
   d. functional units (ref. pg. 31)
9. squamous pneumocyte (ref. pg. 31)
10. granular pneumocyte (ref. pg. 31)
11. 95% (ref. pg. 32)
12. type II (ref. pg. 32)
13. pores of Kohn (ref. pg. 32)
14. alveolar macrophages (ref. pg. 34)
15. tight space, loose space (ref. pg. 34)

SECTION E

1. (ref. pg. 37)
2. resistance (ref. pg. 38)
3. 0.1 μ, 10 μ (ref. pg. 38)
4. capacitance (ref. pg. 39)
5. visceral pleura (ref. pg. 39)
6. loose space of the interstitium (ref. pg. 39)
7. (ref. pg. 41)
8. autonomic nervous system (ref. pg. 40)
9. (ref. pg. 43)
10. epinephrine or norepinephrine (ref. pg. 42)
11. relax (ref. pg. 42)
12. constrict (ref. pg. 42)
13. acetylcholine (ref. pg. 42)

SECTION F

1. first (ref. pg. 42)
2. sixth, eleventh (ref. pgs. 42, 44)
3. hilum (ref. pg. 44)
4. costal, mediastinal (ref. pg. 44)
5. oblique fissure, fourth (ref. pg. 44)
6. costal, mediastinal (ref. pg. 44)
7. (ref. pg. 43)
8. (ref. pg. 44)
9. (ref. pg. 46)
10. trachea, heart, major blood vessels, various nerves, portions of the esophagus, thymus gland, and lymph nodes (ref. pgs. 45, 47)
11. visceral (ref. pg. 47)
12. parietal (ref. pg. 47)
13. pleural cavity (ref. pg. 47)
14. a. manubrium sterni
    b. the body
    c. xyphoid process (ref. pg. 48)
15. true ribs (ref. pg. 48)
16. false (ref. pg. 48)
17. floating (ref. pg. 48)
18. (ref. pg. 49)
19. (ref. pg. 50)

SECTION G

1. central tendon (ref. pg. 48)
2. esophagus, aorta, several nerves, and the inferior vena cava (ref. pg. 48)
3. phrenic (ref. pg. 48)
4. first, second (ref. pg. 51)
5. sternum (ref. pg. 52)
6. chest, anteroposterior (ref. pg. 52)
7. scapula, shoulders, arms (ref. pg. 53)
8. upward, outward (ref. pg. 53)
9. (ref. pg. 58)
10. downward, inward (ref. pgs. 57, 58)

Chapter Two
VENTILATION
Answers

SECTION A

1. driving pressure (ref. pg. 66)
2. transairway pressure (ref. pg. 66)
3. transpulmonary pressure (ref. pg. 66)
4. transthoracic pressure (ref. pg. 68)
5. 5 mm Hg (ref. pg. 66)
6. 7 mm Hg (ref. pg. 66)
7. 6 mm Hg (ref. pg. 66)
8. 6 mm Hg (ref. pg. 68)
9. decrease (ref. pg. 69)
10. greater (ref. pg. 69)
11. below (ref. pg. 69)
12. 3 to 6, 2 to 4 (ref. pgs. 69, 70)
13. study of matter at rest and the forces bringing about or maintaining equilibrium (ref. pg. 70)
14. collapse (ref. pg. 70)
15. expand (ref. pg. 70)
16. 1. the elastic properties of the lung tissue
    2. surface tension produced by the layer of fluid that lines the inside of the alveoli (ref. pg. 71)
17. volume, pressure (ref. pgs. 71, 72)
18.
    - Part I (ref. pgs. 71, 72)
      .055 L/cm H_2O (55 ml/cm H_2O)
    - Part II
      .070 L/cm H_2O (70 ml/cm H_2O)
    - Part III
      Increasing
19.
    - Part I (ref. pgs. 71, 72)
      .050 L/cm H_2O (50 ml/cm H_2O)
    - Part II
      .045 L/cm H_2O (45 ml/cm H_2O)
    - Part III
      decreasing
20. 0.1 L/cm H_2O (ref. pg. 71)
21. 2000 ml (2 liters) (ref. pgs. 71, 72)
22. right (ref. pg. 73)
23. a (ref. pg. 73)
24. b (ref. pg. 73)

SECTION B

1. the natural ability of matter to respond directly to force and to return to its original resting position or shape after the external force no longer exists (ref. pg. 73)
2. the change in pressure per change in volume

   $$\text{Elastance} = \frac{\Delta P}{\Delta V}$$ (ref. pg. 73)

3. low, high (ref. pg. 73)
4. when a truly elastic body, like a spring, is acted on by 1 unit of force, the elastic body will stretch 1 unit of length, and when acted on by 2 units of force it will stretch 2 units of length, and so forth (ref. pg. 73)
5. volume, pressure (ref. pg. 75)
6. surface tension (ref. pg. 75)
7. 70 dynes/cm (ref. pg. 75)
8. $$P = \frac{2ST}{r}$$ (ref. pg. 75)
9. (1) directly proportional to the surface tension of the liquid
   (2) inversely proportional to the radius of the sphere (ref. pg. 77)
10. increases, decreases (ref. pg. 77)
11. b (ref. pg. 77)
12. critical opening pressure (ref. pg. 78)
13. c (ref. pg. 79)
14. alveolar type II cells (ref. pg. 82)
15. water insoluble, water soluble (ref. pg. 82)
16. increases, decrease (ref. pg. 82)
17. 1-5 dynes, 50 dynes (ref. pg. 83)
18. a. acidosis
    b hypoxia
    c. hyperoxia
    d. atelectasis
    e. pulmonary vascular congestion (ref. pg. 85)
19. low (ref. pg. 86)

SECTION C

1. study of forces in action (ref. pg. 86)
2. the movement of in action gas in and out of the lungs and the pressure changes required to move the gas (ref. pg. 86)
3. $$\dot{V} = \frac{\Delta P r^4 \pi}{8 l n}$$ (ref. pg. 86)
4. a. increases
   b. increases
   c. increases
   d. increases (ref. pg. 86)

5. a. 2 liters/min.
   b. 14 liters/minute
   c. 256 cm H_2O
   d. 20 cm H_2O
   e. 800 liters/min.
   f. 200 liters/min
   g. 5 cm H_2O
   h. 2.5 cm H_2O (ref. pgs. 86, 90)

6. $\dot{V} = Pr^4$

   $P = \frac{\dot{V}}{r^4}$ (ref. pg. 90)

7. pressure difference between the mouth and the alveoli divided by flow rate (ref. pg. 91)

8. $R_{aw} = \frac{\Delta P \text{ (cm } H_2O)}{\dot{V} \text{ (L/sec.)}}$ (ref. pg. 92)

9. 3 cm H_2O/L/sec. (ref. pg. 92)

SECTION D

1. 1.0, 2.0 (ref. pg. 92)
2. a gas flow that is streamlined (ref. pg. 93)
3. molecules that move through a tube in a random manner (ref. pg. 93)
4. time (in seconds) necessary to inflate a particular lung region to 60 percent of its potential filling capacity (ref. pg. 93)
5. b (ref. pgs. 93, 94)
6. b (ref. pgs. 93, 94)
7. c (ref. pgs. 93, 94)
8. a (ref. pgs. 93, 94)
9. a (ref. pgs. 93, 94)
10. e (ref. pgs. 93, 94)
11. change in the volume of the lungs divided by the change in the transpulmonary pressure during the time required for one breath (ref. pg. 94)
12. equal to (ref. pg. 94)
13. decreases (ref. pg. 94)
14. alveoli distal to an obstruction that do not have enough time to fill to their potential filling capacity as the breathing frequency increases (ref. pgs. 94, 96)

SECTION E

1. a. tidal volume
   b. ventilatory rate
   c. time relationship between inhalation and exhalation (ref. pg. 96)
2. 7 to 9, 3 to 4 (ref. pg. 96)
3. 15 (ref. pg. 96)
4. 1:2 (ref. pg. 96)
5. alveolar ventilation (ref. pg. 97)
6. deadspace ventilation (ref. pg. 98)
7. the volume of gas in the conducting airways: The nose, mouth, pharynx, larynx and lower airways down to, but not including, the respiratory bronchioles (ref. pg. 98)
8. 130 ml (ref. pg. 98)
9. tidal volume, deadspace ventilation, breaths per minute (ref. pg. 100)
10. 6,240 ml (ref. pg. 100)
11. an alveolus that is ventilated but not perfused with pulmonary blood (ref. pg. 101)
12. the sum of the anatomic deadspace and alveolar deadspace (ref. pg. 101)
13. greater (ref. pgs. 101, 102)
14. greater (ref. pgs. 101, 102)
15. c (ref. pgs. 101, 102)
16. increases, decreases (ref. pg. 102)
17. decreases, increases (ref. pg. 102)
18. energy, ventilation (ref. pg. 102)
19. complete absence of spontaneous ventilation (ref. pg. 105)
20. normal, spontaneous breathing (ref. pg. 106)
21. short episodes of rapid, uniformly deep inspirations, followed by 10 to 30 seconds of apnea (ref. pg. 106)
22. increased depth of breathing with or without an increased frequency (ref. pg. 106)
23. an increased alveolar ventilation produced by any ventilatory pattern that causes the PA_{CO_2} and, therefore, the Pa_{CO_2} to decrease (ref. pg. 107)
24. a decreased alveolar ventilation produced by any ventilatory pattern that causes the PA_{CO_2} and, therefore, the Pa_{CO_2} to increase (ref. pg. 107)
25. a rapid breathing rate (ref. pg. 107)
26. 10 to 30 seconds of apnea, followed by a gradual increase in the volume and frequency of breathing, followed by a gradual decrease in the volume of breathing until another period of apnea occurs (ref. pg. 108)
27. both an increased depth and rate of breathing (ref. pg. 109)
28. a condition in which an individual is able to breathe most comfortably in the upright position (ref. pg. 109)
29. difficulty in breathing, of which the individual is consciously aware (ref. pg. 109)

Chapter Three
THE DIFFUSION OF PULMONARY GASES
Answers

SECTION A

1. the movement of gas molecules from an area of relatively high concentration of gas to one of low concentration (ref. pg. 117)
2. if temperature remains constant, pressure will vary inversely to volume (ref. pg. 118)
3. $P_1 \times V_1 = P_2 \times V_2$ (ref. pg. 118)
4. 66.66 cm H_2O (ref. pg. 118)
5. 37.5 cm H_2O (ref. pg. 118)
6. if pressure remains constant, volume and temperature will vary directly (ref. pg. 118)
7. $V_1/T_1 = V_2/T_2$ (ref. pg. 118)
8. 9.37 L (ref. pg. 118)
9. 4.64 L (ref. pg. 118)
10. if the volume remains constant, pressure and temperature will vary directly (ref. pg. 119)
11. $P_1/T_1 = P_2/T_2$ (ref. pg. 119)
12. 15.62 cm H_2O (ref. pg. 119)
13. 44.53 cm H_2O (ref. pg. 119)
14. in a mixture of gases, the total pressure is equal to the sum of the partial pressures of each separate gas (ref. pg. 119)
15. 650 mm Hg (ref. pg. 119)

SECTION B

1. (ref. pg. 120)
2. decreases, remains the same (ref. pg. 120)
3. (ref. pg. 121)
4. the alveolar oxygen must mix - or compete in terms of partial pressures - with alveolar CO_2 pressure and alveolar water vapor pressure (ref. pg. 121)
5. 44 mg/L, 47 mm Hg (ref. pg. 122)
6. 428.2 mm Hg (ref. pg. 122)

SECTION C

1.
   a. liquid lining the intra-alveolar membrane
   b. alveolar epithelial cell
   c. basement membrane of the alveolar epithelial cell
   d. loose connective tissue (the interstitial space)
   e. basement membrane of the capillary endothelium
   f. capillary endothelium
   g. plasma in the capillary blood
   h. erythrocyte membrane
   i. intracellular fluid in the erythrocyte (ref. pg. 123)

2. 0.36 to 2.5 μ (ref. pg. 123)
3. 40, 46 (ref. pg. 123)
4. 60, 6 (ref. pg. 123)
5. 0.25 (ref. pg. 123)
6. 0.75, one-third (ref. pg. 123)
7. b (ref. pg. 123)
8. $\dot{V}\text{ gas} = \frac{AD(P_1 - P_2)}{T}$ (ref. pg. 124)
9. I. a
   II. a
   III. b (ref. pg. 124)
10. the amount of gas that dissolves in a liquid at a given temperature is proportional to the partial pressure of the gas (ref. pg. 125)
11. solubility coefficient (ref. pg. 125)
12. (1) directly proportional to the solubility coefficient of the gas
    (2) inversely proportional to the square root of the gram-molecular weight of the gas (ref. pg. 129)
13. the transfer of gas across the alveolar wall is a function of the amount of blood that flows past the alveoli (ref. pg. 131)
14. the movement of gas across the alveolar wall is a function of the integrity of the alveolar-capillary membrane itself (ref. pg. 131)
15. a (ref. pgs. 132, 136)

Chapter Four
PULMONARY FUNCTION MEASUREMENTS
Answers

SECTION A

1. the volume of air that normally moves into and out of the lungs in one quiet breath (ref. pg. 141)
2. the maximum volume of air that can be inhaled after a normal tidal volume inhalation (ref. pg. 141)
3. the maximum volume of air that can be exhaled after a normal tidal volume exhalation (ref. pg. 141)
4. the amount of air remaining in the lungs after a maximal exhalation (ref. pg. 141)
5. the maximum volume of air that can be exhaled after a maximal inspiration (ref. pgs. 141, 142)
6. the volume of air that can be inhaled after a normal exhalation (ref. pg. 142)
7. the volume of air remaining in the lungs after a normal exhalation (ref. pg. 142)
8. maximum amount of air that the lungs can accommodate (ref. pg. 142)
9. the percentage of the TLC occupied by the RV (ref. pg. 142)
10. (ref. pg. 143)
11. RV, V_T, FRC, RV/TLC ratio; VC, IC, IRV, ERV (ref. pg. 142)
12. VC, IC, RV, FRC, V_T, TLC (ref. pg. 142)

SECTION B

1. the maximum volume of gas that can be exhaled as forcefully and rapidly as possible after a maximal inspiration (ref. pg. 143)
2. the maximum volume of gas that can be exhaled over a specific period of time (ref. pgs. 143, 144)
3. a. 60%
   b. 83%
   c. 94%
   d. 97% (ref. pg. 144)
4. decreases (ref. pg. 144)
5. the average rate of airflow between 200 and 1200 ml of the FVC (ref. pg. 144)
6. large (ref. pg. 144)
7. the average flow rate during the middle 50 percent of an FVC measurement (ref. pg. 149)
8. medium, small (ref. pg. 149)
9. the maximum flow rate that can be achieved (ref. pg. 149)
10. the largest volume of gas that can be breathed voluntarily in and out of the lungs in 1 minute (ref. pg. 149)

11. the ratio of the volume of gas that can be forcefully exhaled in 1 second to the total volume of gas that can be forcefully exhaled after a maximum inspiration (ref. pg. 149)
12. (ref. pg. 151)
13. (ref. pg. 154)
14. the initial flow rate during forced expiration depends on the muscular effort produced by the individual (ref. pg. 151)
15. once a maximum flow rate has been attained, the flow rate cannot be increased by further muscular effort (ref. pg. 152)
16. dynamic compression (ref. pg. 152)
17. toward the alveolus (upstream) (ref. pg. 153)
18. increases (ref. pg. 153)

Chapter Five
THE CIRCULATORY SYSTEM
Answers

SECTION A

1. a. plasma
   b. erythrocytes
   c. leukocytes
   d. thrombocytes (ref. pg. 162)
2. erythrocytes (ref. pg. 162)
3. 5 (ref. pg. 162)
4. 4 (ref. pg. 162)
5. hematocrit (ref. pg. 162)
6. a. 45%
   b. 42%
   c. 45 to 60% (ref. pgs. 162, 164)
7. 7.5 μ, 2.5 μ (ref. pg. 164)
8. 120 (ref. pg. 164)
9. Protect the body against the invasion of bacteria and other foreign agents that can harm the body (ref. pg. 164)
10. 5,000 to 9,000 (ref. pg. 164)
11. (ref. pg. 164)
12. neutrophils (ref. pg. 164)
13. eosinophils (ref. pgs. 164, 165)
14. monocytes (ref. pg. 165)
15. lymphocytes (ref. pg. 165)
16. platelets (ref. pg. 165)
17. 250,000 and 500,000 (ref. pg. 165)
18. prevent blood loss from a traumatized surface of the body involving the smallest vessels (ref. pg. 165)
19. 55 (ref. pg. 165)
20. 90 (ref. pg. 165)
21. a. albumins
    b. globulins
    c. fibrinogen (ref. pg. 166)
22. a. Na^+
    b. K^+
    c. Ca_2^+
    d. Mg_2^+ (ref. pg. 166)
23. a. Cl^-
    b. PO_4^{3-}
    c. SO_4^{2-}
    d. HCO_3^- (ref. pg. 166)

24. a. amino acids
    b. glucose/carbohydrates
    c. lipids
    d. individual vitamins (ref. pg. 166)
25. a. urea
    b. creatinine
    c. uric acid
    d. bilirubin (ref. pg. 166)

SECTION B

1. (ref. pg. 167)
2. inferior and superior vena cava (ref. pg. 166)
3. tricuspid valve (ref. pg. 166)
4. papillary muscles (ref. pg. 166)
5. pulmonary trunk, pulmonary arteries (ref. pg. 166)
6. pulmonary veins (ref. pg. 166)
7. mitral valve (ref. pg. 166)
8. aorta (ref. pgs. 166, 167)
9. aortic semilunar (ref. pg. 167)
10. (ref. pg. 168)
11. sinoatrial node (ref. pg. 169)
12. sympathetic (ref. pg. 170)
13. parasympathetic (ref. pg. 170)
14. depolarization of the atria (ref. pg. 170)
15. ventricular depolarization (ref. pg. 170)
16. ventricular repolarization (ref. pg. 170)
17. (ref. pg. 172)

SECTION C

1. 60-100 beats/minute (ref. pg. 170)
2. 130 to 140 beats/minute (ref. pg. 170)
3. pulmonary trunk, left atrium (ref. pg. 170)
4. aorta, right atrium (ref. pg. 170)
5. away from (ref. pg. 170)
6. arterioles (ref. pg. 170)
7. arterioles (ref. pgs. 170, 172)
8. arterioles (ref. pg. 172)
9. external (ref. pg. 172)
10. internal (ref. pg. 172)
11. venules (ref. pg. 172)
12. capacitance (ref. pg. 172)
13. 60 (ref. pg. 172)
14. sympathetic (ref. pg. 172)
15. vasomotor, medulla oblongata, sympathetic (ref. pg. 172)
16. sympathetic (ref. pg. 172)
17. vasomotor tone (ref. pg. 172)
18. increasing, sympathetic (ref. pg. 174)
19. decreasing, sympathetic (ref. pg. 174)

20. a. heart
    b. brain
    c. skeletal muscles (ref. pg. 174)
21. pressoreceptors (ref. pg. 174)
22. glossopharyngeal (ref. pg. 175)
23. vagus (ref. pg. 175)
24. decrease, increase (ref. pg. 176)
25. a. an increased cardiac output
    b. an increase in the total peripheral resistance
    c. the return of blood pressure toward normal (ref. pg. 176)
26. a. large arteries
    b. large veins
    c. pulmonary vessels
    d. cardiac walls (ref. pg. 176)

SECTION D

1. actual blood pressure in the lumen of any vessel at any point relative to the barometric pressure (ref. pg. 177)
2. difference between the pressure in the lumen of a vessel and the pressure surrounding the vessel (ref. pg. 177)
3. greater than (ref. pg. 177)
4. less than (ref. pg. 177)
5. pressure difference between the pressure at one point in a vessel and the pressure at any other point downstream in the vessel (ref. pg. 177)
6. systolic pressure (ref. pg. 178)
7. diastolic pressure (ref. pg. 178)
8. 10 (ref. pg. 178)
9. (ref. pg. 180)
10. 40 ml and 80 ml (ref. pgs. 179, 180)
11. cardiac output (ref. pg. 180)
12. 4,400 ml (ref. pg. 180)
13. a (ref. pgs. 180, 181)
14. 5 (ref. pg. 181)
15. 75, 15, 10 (ref. pg. 181)
16. 60, 10 (ref. pg. 182)

SECTION E

1. to the portion of the body, or portion of the organ, that is closest to the ground (ref. pg. 182)
2. greater than (ref. pg. 183)
3. a. posterior
   b. anterior
   c. lung nearest the ground
   d. apexes (ref. pg. 183)
4. alveolar, greater than (ref. pg. 183)
5. a. severe hemorrhage
   b. dehydration
   c. positive pressure ventilation (ref. pg. 183)
6. alveolar dead space (ref. pg. 183)

7. greater than, greater than (ref. pg. 183)
8. greater than, greater than (ref. pg. 184)
9. a. ventricular preload
   b. ventricular afterload
   c. myocardial contractility (ref. pg. 185)
10. the degree the myocardial fiber is stretched prior to contraction (ref. pg. 185)
11. more (ref. pg. 185)
12. ventricular end-diastolic pressure (ref. pg. 186)
13. ventricular end-diastolic volume (ref. pg. 186)
14. a (ref. pg. 186)
15. Frank-Starling Relationship (ref. pg. 186)
16. the force against which the ventricles must work to pump blood (ref. pg. 186)
17. a. the volume and viscosity of blood ejected
    b. peripheral vascular resistance
    c. total cross-sectional area of the vascular space into which blood is ejected (ref. pg. 186)
18. arterial systolic blood pressure (ref. pg. 186)
19. BP = CO x SVR (ref. pg. 186)
20. the force generated by the myocardium when the ventricular muscle fibers shorten (ref. pg. 186)
21. b (ref. pg. 186)
22. a. pulse
    b. blood pressure
    c. skin temperature
    d. serial hemodynamic measurements (ref. pg. 186)
23. positive inotropism (ref. pg. 186)
24. negative inotropism (ref. pg. 186)
25. resistance = $\frac{\text{Mean Blood Pressure}}{\text{Cardiac Output}}$ (ref. pg. 187)
26. a (ref. pg. 188)

SECTION F

1. the physiologic, pharmacologic, or pathologic processes that have a direct effect on the vascular system (ref. pg. 188)
2. a (ref. pg. 188)
3. a (ref. pg. 188)
4. a (ref. pg. 188)
5. a (ref. pg. 188)
6. a. epinephrine (Adrenalin)
   b. norepinephrine (Levophed)
   c. dobutamine (Dobutrex)
   d. dopamine (Intropin)
   e. phenylephrine (Neo-Synephrine) (ref. pg. 189)
7. a. oxygen
   b. isoproterenol (Isuprel)
   c. aminophylline
   d. calcium blocking agents (ref. pg. 189)

8. a. vessel blockage or obstruction
   b. vessel wall diseases
   c. vessel destruction or obliteration
   d. vessel compression (ref. pg. 189)

SECTION G

1. a secondary change in pulmonary vascular resistance that occurs in response to another mechanical change (ref. pg. 189)
2. b (ref. pgs. 189, 190)
3. the opening of vessels that were closed, the stretching or widening of vessels that were open (ref. pg. 190)
4. b (ref. pg. 190)
5. high (ref. pg. 191)
6. low (ref. pg. 192)
7. low (ref. pg. 191)
8. high (ref. pg. 192)
9. low (ref. pg. 192)
10. high (ref. pg. 192)
11. b (ref. pg. 193)
12. a (ref. pg. 194)

Chapter Six
HEMODYNAMIC MEASUREMENTS
Answers

SECTION A

1. the study of the forces that influence the circulation of blood (ref. pg. 201)
2. (ref. pg. 203)
3. (ref. pg. 203)

SECTION B

1. the volume of blood ejected by the ventricles with each contraction (ref. pg. 201)
2. a. preload
   b. afterload
   c. myocardial contractility (ref. pg. 201)
3. $SV = \frac{CO}{HR}$ (ref. pg. 201)
4. 63.21 ml/beat (ref. pg. 202)
5. dividing the stroke volume (SV) by the body surface area (BSA) (ref. pg. 203)
6. 22 ml/beat/m^2 (ref. pg. 204)
7. a. contractility of the heart
   b. overall blood volume status
   c. degree of venous return (ref. pg. 204)
8. dividing the cardiac output (CO) by the body's surface area (BSA) (ref. pg. 205)
9. 2.8 L/minute/m^2 (ref. pg. 205)
10. the amount of work required by the right ventricle to pump blood (ref. pg. 205)
11. contractility of the right ventricle (ref. pg. 205)
12. $RVSWI = SVI \times (\overline{PA} - CVP) \times 0.0136$ gm/ml (ref. pg. 205)
13. 8.16 g m/m^2 (ref. pg. 205)
14. the amount of work required by the left ventricle to pump blood (ref. pg. 206)
15. contractility of the left ventricle (ref. pg. 206)
16. $LVSWI = SVI \times (MAP - PCWP) \times 0.0136$ gm/ml (ref. pg. 206)
17. 70.38 g m/m^2 (ref. pg. 206)
18. (ref. pg. 204)
19. low (ref. pg. 206)
20. high (ref. pg. 206)
21. the afterload of the right ventricle (ref. pg. 206)

22. PVR = $\frac{\overline{PA} - PCWP}{CO}$ X 80 (ref. pg. 206)
23. 114 dynes x sec cm^{-5} (ref. pg. 207)
24. (ref. pg. 207)
25. (ref. pg. 208)
26. the afterload of the left ventricle (ref. pg. 208)
27. SVR = $\frac{MAP - CVP}{CO}$ X 80 (ref. pg. 208)
28. 1266 dynes x sec cm^{-5} (ref. pg. 209)
29. (ref. pg. 208)

CHAPTER SEVEN
OXYGEN TRANSPORT
ANSWERS

SECTION A

1. (ref. pg. 214)

Blood gas	Arterial	Venous
pH	7.35-7.45	7.30-7.40
P_{CO_2}	35-45 mm Hg	42-48 mm Hg
HCO_3^-	22-28 mEq/L	24-30 mEq/L
P_{O_2}	80-100 mm Hg	35-45 mm Hg

2. maintains its precise molecular structure and freely moves throughout the plasma in its normal gaseous state (ref. pg. 214)
3. dissolved O_2 (ref. pg. 214)
4. PART I: 0.15
   PART II: 0.15 Vol% (ref. pg. 214)
5. the amount of O_2 in ml that is in 100 ml of blood (ref. pg. 214)
6. 280 (ref. pg. 215)
7. A (ref. pg. 215)
8. four (ref. pg. 215)
9. $Hb + O_2 \rightleftarrows HbO_2$ (ref. pg. 215)
10. 50, 25 (ref. pg. 216)
11. oxyhemoglobin (ref. pg. 216)
12. reduced hemoglobin or deoxyhemoglobin (ref. pg. 216)
13. directly (ref. pg. 216)
14. two identical α chains, each with 141 amino acids, and two identical β chains, each with 146 amino acids ($\alpha_2 \beta_2$) (ref. pg. 216)
15. two α, two v (ref. pg. 216)
16. methemoglobin (ref. pg. 216)
17. a. 14-16
    b. 12-15
    c. 14-20 (ref. pg. 216)
18. 33 (ref. pg. 216)
19. 1.34 (ref. pg. 216)

20. a. Thebesian venous drainage into the left atrium
    b. bronchial venous drainage into the pulmonary veins
    c. alveoli that are underventilated in proportion to pulmonary blood flow (ref. pg. 217)

SECTION B

1. <u>CASE A</u>
   Question 1: 0.165
   Question 2: 14.807
   Question 3: 14.972
   Question 4: 149.72
   Question 5: 898.32 (ref. pgs. 217, 218)
   <u>CASE B</u>
   Question 1: 0.15
   Question 2: 19.296
   Question 3: 19.446
   Question 4: 194.46
   Question 5: 680.61
   Question 6: 12.135
   Question 7: 24.57 (ref. pgs. 217, 218)

SECTION C

1. percentage, pressure (ref. pg. 218)
2. a. the hemoglobin has an excellent safety zone for the loading of oxygen in the lungs
   b. the diffusion of oxygen during the transit time hemoglobin is in the alveolar-capillary system is enhanced
   c. increasing the P_{O_2} beyond 100 mm Hg adds very little additional oxygen to the blood (ref. pgs. 219, 220)
3. a. P_{O_2} reductions below 60 mm Hg indicate a rapid decrease in the amount of oxygen bound to hemoglobin
   b. a large amount of oxygen is released from the hemoglobin for only a small decrease in P_{O_2} (ref. pg. 220)
4. a. 85%
   b. 17 Vol% (ref. pgs. 218, 221)
5. the partial pressure at which the hemoglobin is 50% saturated with oxygen (ref. pg. 220)
6. 27 (ref. pg. 220)
7. a (ref. pg. 220)
8. b (ref. pg. 220)
9. a. ↑ pH
   ↓ P_{CO_2}
   ↓ Temperature
   ↓ DPG
   HbF
   COHb (ref. pgs. 220, 223)

b. ↓ pH
↑ P_{CO_2}
↑ Temperature
↑ DPG (ref. pgs. 220, 223)
10. b (ref. pg. 224)
11. a (ref. pg. 224)
12 a (ref. pg. 224)
13. b (ref. pg. 224)

SECTION D

1. a. total oxygen delivery
   b. arterial-venous oxygen content difference
   c. oxygen consumption
   d. oxygen extraction ratio
   e. mixed venous oxygen saturation
   f. pulmonary shunting (ref. pg. 231)
2. a. body's ability to oxygenate blood
   b. hemoglobin concentration
   c. cardiac output (ref. pg. 231)

3. $DO_2 = Q_T \times (Ca_{O_2} \times 10)$ (ref. pg. 231)
4. 420 ml O_2/minute (ref. pg. 231)
5. a. decline in blood oxygenation
   b. decline in hemoglobin concentration
   c. decline in cardiac output (ref. pg. 231)

6. between the Ca_{O_2} and the $C\bar{v}_{O_2}$ (ref. pg. 232)

7. $C(a-\bar{v})_{O_2} = Ca_{O_2} - C\bar{v}_{O_2}$ (ref. pg. 233)

8. 4 Vol% (ref. pg. 233)
9. a. decreased cardiac output
   b. periods of increased oxygen consumption
      1) exercise
      2) seizures
      3) shivering post-operative patient
      4) hyperthermia (ref. pg. 233)
10. a. increased cardiac output
    b. skeletal relaxation
    c. peripheral shunting
    d. certain poisons (cyanide)
    e. hypothermia (ref. pg. 234)
11. oxygen consumption, oxygen uptake (ref. pg. 233)

12. $\dot{V}_{O_2} = Q_T[C(a-\bar{v})_{O_2} \times 10]$ (ref. pg. 233)

13. 600 ml O_2/min (ref. pg. 234)

14. a. exercise
    b. seizures
    c. shivering in postoperative patient
    d. hyperthermia (ref. pg. 234)
15. a. skeletal relaxation
    b. peripheral shunting
    c. certain poisons (cyanide)
    d. hypothermia (ref. pg. 235)
16. body surface area (BSA) (ref. pg. 234)
17. 125, 165 (ref. pg. 234)
18. extracted by the peripheral tissues divided by the amount of oxygen delivered to the peripheral cells (ref. pg. 235)
19. a. oxygen coefficient ratio
    b. oxygen utilization ratio (ref. pg. 235)
20. $O_2ER = \frac{Ca_{O_2} - Cv_{O_2}}{Ca_{O_2}}$ (ref. pg. 235)
21. 25 (ref. pg. 235)
22. PART I: 50 (ref. pg. 235)
    PART II: 425, 425 (ref. pg. 235)
23. a. decreased cardiac output
    b. period of increased oxygen consumption
        1. exercise
        2. seizures
        3. shivering in postoperative patient
        4. hyperthermia
    c. anemia
    d. decreased arterial oxygenation (ref. pg. 236)
24. a. increased cardiac output
    b. peripheral shunting
    c. certain poisons (cyanide)
    d. hypothermia
    e. increased hemoglobin concentration
    f. increased arterial oxygenation (ref. pg. 236)
25. 75 (ref. pg. 237)
26. 65 (ref. pg. 237)
27. a. decreased cardiac output
    b. periods of increased oxygen consumption
        1. exercises
        2. seizures
        3. shivering in postoperative patient
        4. hyperthermia (ref. pg. 237)
28. a (ref. pg. 237)

29. a. increased cardiac output
    b. skeletal relaxation
    c. peripheral shunting
    d. certain poisons (cyanide)
    e. hypothermia (ref. pg. 237)
30. b (ref. pg. 237)
31. (ref. pg. 238)

SECTION E

1. that portion of the cardiac output that enters the left side of the heart without exchanging gases with the alveolar gases - or the blood that does exchange gases with alveolar gases but does not obtain a P_{O_2} that equals the alveolus (ref. pg. 238)
2. a. anatomic shunts
   b. capillary shunts (ref. pg. 238)
3. blood flows from the right side of the heart to the left side without coming in contact with an alveolus for gas exchange (ref. pg. 238)
4. 2, 5 (ref. pg. 238)
5. a. congenital heart disease
   b. intrapulmonary fistula
   c. vascular lung tumors (ref. pg. 240)
6. a. alveolar collapse or atelectasis
   b. alveolar fluid accumulation
   c. alveolar consolidation (ref. pg. 240)
7. true, absolute shunt (ref. pg. 240)
8. the hypoxemia produced by an absOolute shunt cannot be treated by simply increasing the concentration of inspired oxygen - since the alveoli are unable to accommodate any form of ventilation (ref. pg. 240)
9. pulmonary capillary perfusion is in excess of alveolar ventilation (ref. pg. 240)
10. a. hypoventilation
    b. uneven distribution of ventilation
    c. alveolar-capillary diffusion defects (ref. pg. 240)
11. the mixing of shunted, non-reoxygenated blood with reoxygenated blood distal to the alveoli (ref. pg. 240)
12. $$\frac{\dot{Q}s}{\dot{Q}t} = \frac{Cc_{O_2} - Ca_{O_2}}{Cc_{O_2} - C\bar{v}_{O_2}}$$ (ref. pg. 241)
13. a. 268.1 mm Hg
    b. 14.204 Vol% O_2
    c. 12.389 Vol% O_2
    d. 8.139 Vol% O_2
    e. .29 (ref. pgs. 242, 243)

14. a. reflects normal lung status
    b. reflects an intrapulmonary abnormality
    c. reflects significant intrapulmonary disease and may be life-threatening in patients with limited cardiovascular or central nervous system function
    d. reflects a potentially life-threatening situation--aggressive cardiopulmonary support is generally required (ref. pg. 243)
15. a. questionable perfusion status
    b. decreased myocardial reserve
    c. unstable oxygen consumption demand (ref. pg. 243)
16. the condition in which the Pa_{O_2} and Ca_{O_2} are abnormally low (ref. pg. 244)
17. a. low alveolar P_{O_2}
    b. diffusion impairment
    c. ventilation/perfusion mismatch (ref. pg. 244)
18. a condition in which the oxygen tension in the arterial blood is normal, but the oxygen-carrying capacity of the blood is inadequate (ref. pgs. 244, 245)
19. a. low amount of hemoglobin in the blood
    b. deficiency in the ability for hemoglobin to carry oxygen (ref. pg. 245)
20. a condition in which the arterial blood that reaches the tissue cells may have a normal oxygen tension and content, but the blood is not adequate to meet tissue needs (ref. pg. 245)
21. a. stagnant hypoxia
    b. arterial-venous shunting (ref. pg. 245)
22. any condition that impairs the ability of tissue cells to utilize oxygen (ref. pg. 245)
23. the term used to describe the blue-gray or purplish discoloration seen on the mucous membranes, fingertips, and toes (ref. pg. 246)
24. an increased level of red blood cells (ref. pg. 247)

Chapter Eight
CARBON DIOXIDE TRANSPORT AND ACID BASE BALANCE
Answers

SECTION A

1. a. carbamino compound
   b. bicarbonate
   c. dissolved CO_2
2. a. dissolved CO_2
   b. carbamino - Hb
   c. bicarbonate (ref. pgs. 252, 253, 254)
3. bicarbonate (ref. pg. 253)
4. 63 (ref. pg. 253)
5. (ref. pg. 252)
6. linear (ref. pg. 254)
7. 40, 50 (ref. pg. 254)
8. Haldane effect (ref. pg. 257)

SECTION B

1. charged species (ions) that can conduct a current in solution (ref. pg. 257)
2. substance that is capable of neutralizing both acids and bases without causing an appreciable change in the original pH (ref. pg. 257)
3. dissociates completely into H^+ and an anion (ref. pg. 257)
4. dissociates only partially into ions (ref. pg. 258)
5. dissociates completely (ref. pg. 258)
6. reacts with water to form OH^- in an equilibrium; partial dissociation (ref. pg. 258)
7. weak acid or base systems that have an equilibrium between the molecular form and its ions (ref. pg. 258)
8. [H+] + [A-] (ref. pg. 258)
9. neutral (ref. pg. 259)
10. acidic (ref. pg. 259)
11. basic (ref. pg. 259)
12. the negative logarithm, to the base 10, of the hydrogen ion concentration (ref. pg. 259)
13. $pH = -\log_{10}[H^+]$ (ref. pg. 259)
14. 10^{-7} (ref. pg. 259)
15. donates (ref. pg. 259)
16. decreases (ref. pg. 259)
17. accepts (ref. pg. 259)
18. increases (ref. pg. 259)
19. a. the buffer systems of the blood and tissue
    b. the respiratory ability to regulate the elimination of CO_2
    c. the renal ability to regulate the excretion of hydrogen and reabsorption of bicarbonate ions (ref. pg. 259)
20. carbonic acid/sodium bicarbonate (ref. pg. 260)

21. $pK + \log \frac{[HCO_3^-]}{[H_2CO_3]}$ (ref. pg. 260)
22. the dissociation constant of the acid portion of the buffer combination (ref. pg. 260)
23. 6.1 (ref. pg. 260)
24. 20, 1 (ref. pg. 261)
25. b (ref. pg. 261)
26. c (ref. pg. 261)

SECTION C

1. a. increase
   b. increase
   c. increase
   d. decrease
   e. decrease (ref. pg. 262)
2. d (ref. pgs. 262, 263)
3. a (ref. pgs. 262, 263)
4. a. decreases
   b. decreases
   c. decreases
   d. increases
   e. increases (ref. pgs. 263, 264)
5. a (ref. pgs. 264, 265)
6. b (ref. pgs. 264, 265)
7. false (ref. pg. 265)
8. b (ref. pg. 266)
9. a. lactic acidosis
   b. keto-acidosis
   c. renal failure (ref. pgs. 266, 267)
10. a (ref. pg. 268)
11. a (ref. pg. 268)
12. a. hypokalemia
    b. hypochloremia
    c. gastric suction or vomiting
    d. excessive administration of steroids
    e. excessive administration of sodium bicarbonate (ref. pgs. 268, 269)
13. (ref. pgs. 263-270)
    a. 7.23, 29
    b. 7.58, 17 or 18
    c. Part I: combination of both
       Part II: base deficit
       Part III: 12 to 14 mEq/L
    d. Part I: respiratory
       Part II: base excess
       Part III: 3 to 4 mEq/L

CHAPTER NINE
VENTILATION - PERFUSION RELATIONSHIPS
ANSWERS

SECTION A

1. 4 (ref. pg. 274)
2. 5 (ref. pg. 274)
3. 4:5, 0.8 (ref. pg. 275)
4. higher (ref. pg. 275)
5. lower (ref. pg. 275)
6. decreases (ref. pg. 275)
7. a. the amount of oxygen ventilated into the alveoli
   b. the amount of oxygen removal by capillary blood flow (ref. pg. 276)
8. a. the amount of carbon dioxide that diffuses into the alveoli from the capillary blood
   b. the amount of carbon dioxide removal out of the alveoli by means of ventilation (ref. pg. 276)
9. it washes out of the alveoli faster than it is replaced by the venous blood (ref. pg. 276)
10. it does not diffuse into the blood as fast as it enters the alveolus. The PA_{O_2} also increases because of the reduced PA_{CO_2} (ref. pg. 276, 277)
11. a (ref. pg. 278)
12. oxygen moves out of the alveolus and into the pulmonary capillary blood faster than it is replenished by ventilation (ref. pg. 278)
13. it moves out of the capillary blood and into the alveolus faster than it is washed out of the alveolus (ref. pg. 278)
14. c (ref. pg. 278)
15. decreases (ref. pg. 278)
16. increases (ref. pg. 278)
17. decreases (ref. pg. 278)
18. gas exchange between the systemic capillaries and the tissue cells (ref. pg. 278)
19. 250 (ref. pg. 278)
20. 200 (ref. pg. 281)
21. ratio between the volume of oxygen consumed and the volume of carbon dioxide produced (ref. pg. 281)
22. $RQ = \dfrac{\dot{V}_{CO_2}}{\dot{V}_{O_2}}$ (ref. pg. 281)
23. gas exchange between the pulmonary capillaries and the alveoli (ref. pg. 283)
24. quantity of oxygen and carbon dioxide exchanged during a period of one minute (ref. pg. 283)

25. a. pulmonary emboli
    b. partial or complete obstruction in the pulmonary artery or arterioles
    c. extrinsic pressure on the pulmonary vessels
    d. destruction of the pulmonary vessels
    e. decreased cardiac output (ref. pg. 284)
26. a. obstructive lung disorder
    b. restrictive lung disorders
    c. hypoventilation from any cause (ref. pg. 284)

CHAPTER TEN
CONTROL VENTILATION
ANSWERS

SECTION A

1. a. Dorsal Respiratory Group
   b. Ventral Respiratory Group (ref. pg. 287)
2. a (ref. pg. 287)
3. c (ref. pg. 287)
4. b. VRG (ref. pg. 287)
5. the middle and lower pons (ref. pg. 288)
6. b (ref. pg. 288)
7. b (ref. pg. 288)
8. hydrogen ions [H^+] (ref. pg. 289)
9. bilaterally and ventrally in the substance of the medulla (ref. pg. 289)
10. CO_2, H^+, HCO_3^- (ref. pg. 290)
11. $CO_2 + H_2O \rightleftharpoons H_2CO_3 \rightleftharpoons H^+ + HCO_3^-$ (ref. pg. 290)
12. The central chemoreceptors transmit signals to the respiratory component in the medulla, which, in turn, increases alveolar ventilation (ref. pg. 290)
13. indirect, pH level of the CSF (ref. pg. 290)
14. special oxygen-sensitive cells that react to reductions of oxygen levels in the arterial blood (ref. pg. 290)
15. High in neck at the bifurcation of the internal and external carotid arteries and on the aortic arch (ref. pg. 290)
16. glossopharyngeal (9th); vagus (10th) (ref. pg. 290)
17. a (ref. pg. 290)
18. 60 mm Hg (ref. pg. 290)
19. 30 mm Hg (ref. pg. 291)
20. A chronically high CO_2 concentration in the CSF inactivates the H^+ sensitivity of the central chemoreceptors. HCO_3^- moves into the CSF via the active transport mechanism and combines with H^+, thus returning the pH to normal (ref. pg. 291)
21. a (ref. pg. 291)
22. a. chronic anemia
    b. carbon monoxide poisoning
    c. methemoglobinemia (ref. pg. 292)
23. a. decreased pH (↑ H^+ level)
    b. hypoperfusion
    c. increased temperature
    d. nicotine
    e. the direct effect of Pa_{CO_2} (ref. pgs. 292, 293, 294)

24. a. peripheral vasoconstriction
    b. increased pulmonary vascular resistance
    c. systemic arterial hypertension
    d. tachycardia
    e. increase in left ventricular performance (ref. pg. 294)

SECTION B

1. lung overinflation (ref. pg. 297)
2. inspiration to cease (ref. pg. 297)
3. lung compression or deflation (ref. pg. 297)
4. an increased rate of breathing (ref. pgs. 297, 298)
5. lung compression, or lung exposure to noxious gases (ref. pg. 298)
6. the trachea, bronchi, and bronchioles (ref. pg. 298)
7. the ventilatory rate to increase (ref. pg. 298)
8. in the interstitial tissues between the pulmonary capillaries and the alveoli (ref. pg. 298)
9. a. pulmonary capillary congestion
   b. capillary hypertension
   c. edema of the alveolar walls
   d. humoral agents (serotonin)
   e. lung deflation
   f. emboli (ref. pg. 298)
10. rapid, shallow breathing (ref. pg. 298)
11. a decreased heart and ventilatory rate (ref. pg. 298)
12. an increased heart and ventilatory rate (ref. pg. 298)
13. a. may cause respirations to temporarily cease
    b. may cause a temporary cessation of breathing
    c. can cause an immediate cessation of breathing, followed by an episode of coughing
    d. triggers an increased respiratory rate
    e. may increase ventilation (ref. pgs. 298, 299)

CHAPTER ELEVEN
CARDIOPULMONARY PHYSIOLOGY OF THE FETUS AND THE NEWBORN
ANSWERS

SECTION A

1. a. embryonic
   b. pseudoglandular
   c. canalicular
   d. terminal sac (ref. pg. 304)
2. 24th (ref. pg. 304)
3. 20 (ref. pg. 304)
4. 28th (ref. pg. 306)
5. cotyledons (ref. pg. 306)
6. (ref. pg. 308)
7. umbilical arteries (ref. pg. 306)
8. 20, 55 (ref. pg. 306)
9. the decreased maternal P_{CO_2} is caused by the alveolar hyperventilation that develops as the growing infant restricts the mother's diaphragmatic excursion (ref. pg. 306)
10. a. maternal-fetal P_{O_2} gradient
    b. higher hemoglobin concentration in the fetal blood
    c. greater affinity of fetal hemoglobin for oxygen (ref. pgs. 306, 307)
11. 30, 40 (ref. pg. 307)
12. umbilical vein (ref. pgs. 307, 308)
13. a. the placenta itself is an actively metabolizing organ
    b. the permeability of the placenta varies from region to region with respect to respiratory gases
    c. the fetal and maternal vascular shunts (ref. pgs. 308, 309)

SECTION B

1. ductus venosus (ref. pg. 309)
2. foramen ovale (ref. pg. 309)
3. left ventricle, heart, brain (ref. pg. 309)
4. ductus arteriosus, aorta (ref. pg. 309)
5. 15, pulmonary veins (ref. pg. 309)
6. 20 (ref. pg. 309)

MATCHING:

7. 1. E
   2. C
   3. A
   4. B
   5. D (ref. pg. 309)
8. a. the placenta is passed by the mother
   b. the umbilical arteries atrophy and become the lateral umbilical ligaments
   c. the umbilical vein becomes the round ligament (ligamentum teres) of the liver
   d. the ductus venosus becomes the lagamentum venosum, which is a fibrous cord in the liver
   e. the flap on the foramen ovale usually closes and becomes a depression in the interatrial septum called the Fossa Ovalis
   f. the ductus arteriosus atrophies and becomes the ligamentum arteriosum (ref. pg. 309)

SECTION C

1. a. about one-third of the fluid is squeezed out of the lungs as the infant passes through the birth canal
   b. about one-third of the fluid is absorbed by the pulmonary capillaries
   c. about one-third of the fluid is removed by the lymphatic system (ref. pg. 311)
2. 24 (ref. pg. 311)
3. 12 (ref. pg. 311)
4. a. thermal
   b. tactile
   c. visual (ref. pg. 311)
5. -40 (ref. pg. 311)
6. 40 (ref. pg. 311)
7. .005 L/cm H_2O (ref. pg. 313)
8. 30 cm H_2O/L/sec (ref. pg. 313)
9. a. the sudden increase in the alveolar P_{O_2}, which offsets the hypoxic vasoconstriction
   b. the mechanical increase in lung volume, which widens the caliber of the extra-alveolar vessels (ref. pg. 313)
10. as the pulmonary vascular resistance decreases, a greater amount of blood flows through the lungs, and therefore more blood returns to the left atrium. This causes the pressure in the left atrium to increase and the flap of the foramen ovale to close (ref. pg. 313)
11. 45, 50 (ref. pg. 313)
12. when the ductus arteriosus remains open (permitting blood to pass through it), and the pulmonary vascular resistance is elevated, persistent pulmonary hypertension of the neonate is said to exist. (ref. pg. 313)
13. persistent fetal circulation
14. a. bradykinin
    b. serotonin
    c. prostaglandin inhibitors (ref. pg. 313)

15. peripheral, central (ref. pg. 313)
16. decrease (ref. pg. 314)
17. respiratory slowing or apnea (ref. pgs. 314, 315)
18. marked hyperventilation (ref. pgs. 314, 315)
19. a deep inspiration that is elicited by lung inflation (ref. pg. 316)
20. (ref. pg. 314)
21. (ref. pg. 315)

Chapter Twelve
RENAL FAILURE AND ITS INFLUENCE ON THE CARDIOPULMONARY SYSTEM
Answers

SECTION A

1. (ref. pg. 322)
2. (ref. pg. 323)
3. (ref. pg. 324)

Section B

1. (ref. pg. 326)
2. a. proximal convoluted tubule
   b. loop of Henle
   c. distal convoluted tubule (ref. pg. 325)
3. proximal convoluted tubule (ref. pg. 326)
4. various substances are transported from the plasma of the peri-tubular capillaries to the fluid of the renal tubule (ref. pg. 326)
5. hydrogen (H^+), potassium (K^+) (ref. pg. 326)
6. a. countercurrent mechanism
   b. selective permeability of the collecting duct (ref. pg. 327)
7. renal medulla (ref. pg. 327)
8. 300 (ref. pg. 327)
9. 300, 1,200 (ref. pg. 327)
10. hypothalamus, pituitary gland (ref. pg. 327)
11. b (ref. pg. 327)
12. a (ref. pg. 327)
13. increases (ref. pg. 327)
14. decreases (ref. pg. 327)
15. 1.018 to 1.040 (ref. pg. 327)
16. a. sodium
    b. potassium
    c. calcium, magnesium, and phosphate (ref. pg. 329)
17. hydrogen (ref. pg. 330)
18. sodium bicarbonate (ref. pg. 330)
19. a. capillary fluid shift system
    b. the renal system (ref. pgs. 330, 331)

SECTION C

1. a. unilateral renal agenesis
   b. renal dysplasia
   c. polycystic disease of the kidney (ref. pg. 332)
2. women (ref. pg. 332)
3. a. calculi
   b. normal pregnancy
   c. prostatic hypertrophy
   d. infection and inflammation causing scar tissue
   e. neurologic disorders (ref. pg. 332)
4. a. altered immune responses
   b. drugs and related chemicals
   c. radiation (ref. pgs. 332, 333)
5. Wilms' Tumor (ref. pg. 333)
6. a. hypovolemia
   b. septicemia
   c. heart failure
   d. renal artery atherosclerosis (ref. pg. 333)
7. a sharp reduction in urine output (ref. pg. 333)
8. a. renal ischemia
   b. injury to the glomerular membrane caused by nephrotoxic agents
   c. acute tubular necrosis
   d. intratubular obstruction
   e. acute inflammatory condition (ref. pg. 334)
9. a. ureteral obstruction (ref. pg. 334)
   b. bladder outlet obstruction
10. decreases (ref. pg. 334)
11. increases (ref. pg. 334)
12. a (ref. pg. 334)
13. b (ref. pg. 334)
14. sodium (ref. pg. 335)
15. a. increases
    b. increases
    c. decreases (ref. pgs. 335, 336)
16. b (ref. pgs. 335, 336)
17. b (ref. pgs. 335, 336)
18 a (ref. pgs. 335, 336)
19. a (ref. pgs. 335, 336)
20. a. the production of erythropoietin is often inadequate to stimulate the production of red blood cells
    b. toxic waste accumulation suppresses the ability of bone marrow to produce red blood cells (ref. pg. 336)
21. because of the platelet abnormalities associated with renal failure (ref. pg. 336)
22. this condition develops as a result of the pericardium exposure to the metabolic end-products associated with renal decline (ref. pg. 336)

Chapter Thirteen
AGING AND ITS INFLUENCE ON THE CARDIOPULMONARY S
Answers

SECTION A

1. 20 (ref. pg. 341)
2. 20, 25 (ref. pg. 341)
3. decreases, increases (ref. pg. 342)
4. a. increases
   b. decreases
   c. decreases
   d. remains the same
   e. increases
   f. increases
   g. decreases (ref. pgs. 344, 345)
5. a. decreases
   b. decreases
   c. decreases
   d. decreases
   e. decreases
   f. decreases (ref. pgs. 345, 346)
6. a. decreases (ref. pg. 346)
   b. increases (ref. pg. 346)
   c. increases (ref. pg. 346)
   d. decreases (ref. pgs. 346, 347)
   e. remains the same (ref. pgs. 346, 347)
   f. remains the same (ref. pgs. 346, 347)
   g. remains the same (ref. pgs. 346, 347)
   h. decreases (ref. pg. 347)
   i. decreases (ref. pg. 347)
7. b (ref. pg. 347)
8. b (ref. pg. 347)
9. b (ref. pg. 348)
10. b (ref. pg. 348)
11. b (ref. pgs. 348, 349)
12. 150 (ref. pgs. 348, 349)
13. a. decreases (ref. pgs. 349, 350)
    b. decreases (ref. pg. 350)
    c. increases (ref. pg. 351)
    d. increases (ref. pg. 351)
    e. increases (ref. pg. 351)

Chapter Fourteen
EXERCISE AND ITS EFFECTS ON THE CARDIOPULMONARY SYSTEM
Answers

SECTION A

1.
   a. 20
   b. 3
   c. 6
   d. 25
   e. 20
   f. 20 (ref. pg. 357)
2. 30, 60 (ref. pg. 357)
3. 30, 5 (ref. pg. 357)
4. 40 (ref. pg. 357)
5. Anaerobic Threshold (ref. pg. 357)
6. a. The cerebral cortex sending neural signals to the exercising muscles may also send collateral signals to the medulla to increase the rate and depth of breathing.
   b. Proprioceptors in the moving muscles, tendons, and joints transmit sensory signals via the spinal cord to the respiratory centers of the medulla.
   c. The increase in body temperature during exercise may also contribute to increased ventilation. (ref. pg. 357)

SECTION B

1. e (ref. pg. 357)
2. dept, rate (ref. pg. 358)
3. depth, frequency (rate) (ref. pg. 358)
4. e (ref. pg. 358)
5. a. an increase in alveolar ventilation, within seconds after the onset of exercise.
   b. a slow, gradual further increase in alveolar ventilation developing over approximately the first 3 minutes of exercise.
   c. alveolar ventilation stabilizes. (ref. pg. 358)
6. 50, 65 (ref. pg. 358)

7. 250 (ref. pg. 360)
8. 95 (ref. pg. 360)
9. c (ref. pg. 361)
10. increased cardiac output (ref. pg. 361)
11. d (ref. pg. 362)

SECTION C

1. a. sympathetic discharge
   b. ↑ in cardiac output
   c. ↑ in arterial blood pressure (ref. pg. 363)
2. a. The heart is stimulated to increase its rate and strength of contraction
   b. The blood vessels of the peripheral vascular system constrict, except for the blood vessels of the working muscles, which dilate (ref. pg. 364)
3. an increased cardiac output (ref. pg. 364)
4. a. an increased stroke volume
   b. an increased heart rate
   c. combination of both (ref. pg. 364)
5. vasodilation (ref. pg. 365)
6. Frank-Starling (ref. pg. 365)
7. 165 (ref. pg. 365)
8. increases, decreases (ref. pg. 365)
9. a. the individual's physical condition
   b. the specific muscles that are working
   c. the distribution of blood flow (ref. pg. 365)
10. decreases (ref. pg. 365)
11. a. the sympathetic discharge
    b. the increased cardiac output
    c. the vasoconstriction of the blood vessels in the non-working muscle areas. (ref. pg. 365)
12. a. increases
    b. increases
    c. increases
    d. increases (ref. pg. 365)
13. local vasodilators (ref. pg. 367)
14. heart rate, increased stroke volume (ref. pg. 368)
15. 50 (ref. pg. 369)
16. increased heart rate (ref. pg. 369)
17. 65 (ref. pg. 369)
18. Profuse sweating, followed by no sweating; extreme weakness; muscle cramping; exhaustion; nausea; headache; dizziness; confusion; staggering gait; unconsciousness; circulatory collapse (ref. pg. 370)
19. a. Spraying cool water on the victim's body
    b. Continually sponging the victim with cool water
    c. Blowing air over the body with a strong fan
    d. A combination of all three (ref. pg. 370)
20. a. Acute, inpatient
    b. Outpatient, immediately after hospitalization
    c. Long-term outpatient
    d. Maintenance (ref. pg. 371)

Chapter Fifteen
HIGH ALTITUDE AND ITS EFFECTS ON THE CARDIOPULMONARY SYSTEM
Answers

SECTION A

1. 18,000-19,000 (ref. pg. 375)
2. increased alveolar ventilation (ref. pg. 375)
3. six weeks (ref. pg. 377)
4. c (ref. pg. 377)
5. c (ref. pg. 377)
6. 20-25% greater (ref. pg. 377)
7. a (ref. pg. 377)
8. increased (ref. pgs. 379, 380)
9. c (ref. pg. 380)
10. a (ref. pg. 380)
11. a (ref. pgs. 380, 381)

SECTION B

1. headache, fatigue, dizziness, palpitation, nausea, loss of appetite, and insomnia (ref. pg. 381)
2. second or third day after ascent (ref. pg. 381)
3. vasoconstriction; increased (ref. pg. 381)
4. photophobia, ataxia, hallucinations, clouding of consciousness, coma, and possibly death (ref. pg. 381)
5. fatigue, reduced exercise tolerance, headache, dizziness, somnolence, loss of mental acuity, marked polycythemia, and severe hypoxemia (ref. pg. 382)

Chapter Sixteen
HIGH-PRESSURE ENVIRONMENTS AND THEIR EFFECT ON THE CARDIOPULMONARY SYSTEM
Answers

SECTION A

1. 1.0 atmosphere (ref. pg. 387)
2. PART I: 1.375 liters (ref. pg. 387)
   PART II: 3040 mm Hg (ref. pg. 387)
3. a. the diver's metabolic rate
   b. The diver's ability to store and transport O_2 and CO_2 (ref. pg. 389)
4. 55 (ref. pg. 389)
5. descends, ascends (ref. pgs. 389, 390)
6. hypoxia of ascent (ref. pg. 390)
7. a. bradycardia
   b. decreased cardiac output
   c. peripheral vasoconstriction (ref. pg. 390)
8. a. Joint pains (the bends)
   b. Chest pain and coughing (the chokes)
   c. Paresthesia and paralysis (spinal cord involvement)
   d. Circulatory failure
   e. Death (severe cases) (ref. pg. 390)
9. (ref. pg. 392)
10. a. increases the physically dissolved O_2 in the arterial blood
    b. increases the pressure gradient for driving oxygen into ischemic tissues
    c. reduces the half-life of carboxyhemoglobin (HbCO) (ref. pg. 393)
11. 1 hour (ref. pg. 393)